NURSING .

The Philosophy and Science of Caring

NURSING

JEAN WATSON, R.N., Ph.D.

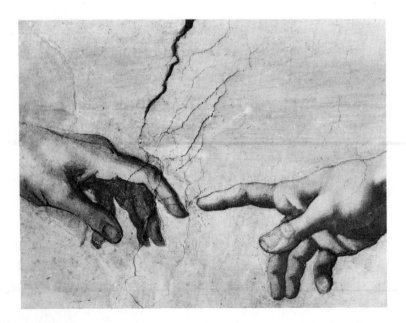

The Philosophy and Science
of Caring

*Dean and Professor, School of Nursing
University of Colorado Health Sciences Center, Denver*

Foreword by Madeleine Leininger

COLORADO ASSOCIATED UNIVERSITY PRESS

Copyright © 1985 by Jean Watson
Published by Colorado Associated University Press
Boulder, Colorado 80309
ISBN 0-87081-154-1
Library of Congress Catalog Card Number 78-71220
Printed in the United States of America
Frontispiece: *Hands of Adam and God* by Michelangelo (Alinari/
Editorial Photocolor archives)

First published by Little, Brown and Company, 1979

Colorado Associated University Press is a cooperative publishing enterprise supported in part by Adams State College, Colorado State University, Fort Lewis College, Mesa College, Metropolitan State College,
University of Colorado, University of Northern Colorado, University of
Southern Colorado, and Western State College

To Doug, Jennifer, and Julie
and to my students

CONTENTS

FOREWORD

In the evolution of the nursing profession, the phrases nursing care, therapeutic care, caring for others, *and related expressions are used by nurses to describe their professional service to others. Members of our society have different thoughts and role expectations about these phrases in relation to the kind of care they receive from nurses. Furthermore, these expressions hold different meanings for nurses in their various care-giving roles, such as to individual clients, families, and community groups they serve. Care-giving and care-receiving roles of nurses have different sets of expectations and behaviors. It is well, therefore, that members of the nursing profession begin systematically to clarify the diverse functions and cultural values related to the concepts of care, caring, and nursing care.*

The concept of care is probably one of the least understood ideas used by professional and nonprofessional people, yet it is probably one of the most important concepts to be understood by human groups. It is a word with multiple social usages in the American culture, and has other meanings in other world cultures. The terms care, caring, *and* nursing care *have both symbolic and functional meanings as they are used by care-givers and care-recipients. Nursing care also has a general, special meaning to nurses, and is often taken for granted in nurses' thoughts and action patterns. It is time that we study the implicit and explicit meanings associated with the concepts of care and caring so that we can reduce their ambiguities. Furthermore, the humanistic, scientific, and linguistic meanings related to nursing care and caring behaviors in any culture remain a most fascinating area of study for nurses.*

From a nursing and anthropological viewpoint, the idea of care for self and others is one of the oldest forms of human expression. Since the beginning of mankind, care appears to be the critical factor in bringing newborns into existence, in stimulating individual growth, and in helping people to survive a variety of stressful experiences. Caring for others has been important in maintaining social alliance, providing psychological support systems, and in bringing about cultural norm satisfactions. Caring for others prompted humans to express their feelings toward others and for individual self-fulfillment. Transcultural aspects of care are barely understood, yet they appear to play a critical role in health maintenance and social relationships within cultural groups.

The nursing profession has long made claims to the concept of care and nursing care. However, nurses have not pursued a systematic investigation of the linguistic, cultural, and psychosocial impact of care-behaviors and processes. Moreover, the concept of care has not been examined from a cross-cultural viewpoint from a folk and a professional point of view.

One of the reasons I have been pursuing cross-cultural studies on caring behaviors and processes is that scientific knowledge of care is limited; and yet, I hold it is the central concept and essence of nursing. Moreover, care is a vital factor for human growth, health maintenance, and survival. Hopefully, as we study the linguistic, cultural, professional, and societal meanings and usages of care, we will discover some entirely new or different aspects of care and the efficacy of its cultural, psychosocial, and physiological modes of helping people. Already, from my preliminary cross-cultural findings about caring processes and behaviors, it is evident that there are divergent meanings and cultural usages related to care-givers and care-recipients. It is further apparent that cultural values and social structure greatly influence the nature, character, and manifestation of care by professional and nonprofessional people. There are also clues that the philosophy, nature, and manifestations of cultural caring have some universal and non-universal features and that care is important for self-growth and self-actualization of cultural groups. Thus, the cross-cultural study of caring behaviors is an enormously rich and important area for professional nurses, especially for nurses prepared in anthropology and psychology who can more readily understand the contextual and ethnological aspects of human behaviors and relationships.

Human caring and human relationships are closely inter-related. Human caring remains an essential dimension of pro-fessional work, especially in dealing with life crises, health maintenance problems, and changes in health practices. *The socialization process of preparing competent, sensitive, and humanistic professional nurses as care-providers is a major challenge for the nursing profession.*

In this book, the author has provided some enormously helpful ideas about the concept of care, with the goal of encouraging the nursing profession to develop a science of caring for nursing practice. *Dr. Watson provides the reader with many seminal, thought-provoking ideas about caring, especially as a therapeutic interpersonal relationship process. The central theme of the author is that caring processes are intrinsic to therapeutic interpersonal relationships between the nurse and client.* She believes that a full understanding and appreciation of caring can come from the behavioral, physical, and social sciences as well as from the humanities, and must be pursued by nurses. *Dr. Watson also contends that a science of caring is essential to the discipline of nursing.* The author helps the reader become actively aware of the concept of care as an important interpersonal process and offers ways to test this knowledge base.

As the author draws upon her nursing and psychology back-ground, she helps the reader to examine the interpersonal aspects of caring in relation to her creatively formulated "cara-tive" factors. These factors serve as structural guides to under-standing the phenomenon of care in an interpersonal relation-ship process. *The basic assumptions and descriptive content are most stimulating, and help one to understand some of the scientific and humanistic aspects of nursing practices as carative forces in human relationships.* Basic human needs — human relationships and the maintenance of health — are linked closely with carative behaviors and processes. *Unques-tionably, caring as a humanistic and interpersonal process is clearly the central theme of this book.*

The author is, therefore, to be commended for offering readers a comprehensive and timely presentation on the sub-ject of caring from an interpersonal perspective. She challenges *the reader with substantive new and refreshing ideas to perceive caring as the integral aspect of all therapeutic nursing practices. This important work contributes to the science of caring. The serious and sensitive nurse who has always valued the importance of caring will be encouraged to see a reaffirmation that care remains central to nursing practices. At the same time, this work encourages the nurse to discover some new insights about humanistic and scientific caring from an interpersonal perspective. It is indeed most encouraging to have this book available to stimulate nurses toward the testing and refinement of the diverse concepts related to caring and nursing care processes. For as our knowledge of caring becomes tested and refined, I predict we shall see a marked, more explicit advancement and improvement in the teaching and practice of therapeutic nursing care.*

Madeleine Leininger, R.N., Ph.D., L.H.D., F.A.A.N.
Professor of Nursing and Anthropology
Director of Center for Health Research
Program Director of Transcultural Nursing
Wayne State University

PREFACE

This book was originally planned as a standard textbook for an integrated undergraduate baccalaureate nursing curriculum. It soon became clear that certain components of an integrated curriculum really comprise basic core processes of nursing. Because those basic processes are so essential to the study of nursing, it would be inhibiting to develop a textbook for an integrated nursing curriculum. It became more challenging and perhaps more useful to develop a new structure for understanding basic nursing processes as the foundation for the science of caring.

A basic examination of the field of nursing reveals great diversity in practice as well as education. The term nursing *is an oversimplification; one could speak instead of professional nursing, technical nursing, and (currently) academic nursing and (or) nursing research. Contemporary nursing is complicated further by the emergence of nurse practitioners and even nurse healers.*

With so much complexity and movement in the nursing field, it is risky to write a book that might have relevance to all of nursing. I have concentrated on nursing "core" rather than on nursing "trim." The term trim *refers to the practice setting, the procedures, the specialized clinical focus, and the techniques and specific terminology surrounding the diverse orientations and preoccupations of nursing. The term* core *refers to those aspects of nursing that are intrinsic to the actual nurse-patient/client process that produces therapeutic results in the person being served. I refer to this basic core of nursing as comprising the philosophy and science of caring.*

If one discards the trim and considers only the process and methods that effect a positive health change in the patient/client, the core is remarkably similar for diverse groups of nurses. Also, the nurses and other health professionals who do not succeed in effecting positive health changes are probably

those who are concerned with trim rather than with core. I
have termed the core mechanisms the carative factors.

When the nursing core is organized according to the carative factors relevant to the philosophy and science of caring,
the whole of nursing seems more comprehensible — more
ordered for understanding and studying. Such organization
also helps to identify the core as the basic foundation for
nursing practice.

Nurses with similar goals use similar carative factors and
effect positive health change in their patient/client. Although
the carative factors are the primary ingredients for effective
nursing practice, the trim of the different groups of nurses is
in no way expendable. Each nurse, depending on her or his
educational background, clinical focus, and personality,
masters an approach to nursing care that enhances the operation of the carative factors. Often the commitment of the
nurse to a particular field of nursing or to particular skills aids
in the initial stages of the nurse–patient/client relationship.
Confidence, trust, faith, and positive expectations are increased.
The patient/client is more likely to value the nurse, to attend
to the communication and behavior more actively, and to participate in the process more completely when the nurse is
confident and competent in delivery of care.

In learning and practice behavior, trim must be distinguished
from core. If the trim (skills, techniques, specialized language,
and so on) is considered to be the critical agent for effecting
positive health change or quality care, the carative factors may
be neglected. The neglect occurs especially when the trim
becomes elaborate and esteemed, and the trim may become
elaborate and esteemed if nursing has difficulty in identifying
and establishing its core.

This book approaches the field of nursing by discussing the
primary carative factors that make up the core. The factors I
describe are not original; they are already used by most nurses.
The term carative factors was suggested by the contrast of
caring with curing knowledge. The curative factors of Yalom*
suggested and helped define the carative factors that comprise

*I. G. Yalom. The Theory, Knowledge and Practice of Group Psychotherapy (2nd
ed.). New York: Basic Books, 1975.

the science and practice of nursing. The concepts, ideas, theories, and findings of research presented in this book need further study, development, and research; but they may help to guide the study of nursing as the science of caring. This book suggests a scientific basis for the carative factors that are essential to effective nursing care.

Nursing is both scientific and artistic. I seek to combine science with humanism; and I view nursing as a therapeutic interpersonal process. That basic, immeasurable, interpersonal aspect is the foundation of the carative factors. At the same time, nursing is a scientific discipline that derives — and must continue to derive — its practice base from scientific knowledge and research. My hope is that the content and structure offered here will help nurses and other health professionals understand and study nursing as a humanistic-scientific discipline as well as an academic-clinical profession.

J. W.

PREFACE TO SECOND PRINTING

I have been heartened and encouraged that the first printing of this book has been labeled by others as a timeless work that needs to remain in print. During the last year, since the book has been sold out and is out of print, I have received numerous and wide-ranging requests for copies and permission to use the work, including permission for foreign translation rights.

Since publication of this book in 1979, it has been studied and researched as a nursing theory and incorporated into several nursing curricula in the United States and other parts of the world. It has been used as a guiding philosophy to incorporate arts and humanities into nursing science. The caring ideas have been examined by master level students in concept development courses. Doctoral students study the work as a theory of nursing. The book has been recommended as a framework which emphasizes the interrelationship between nurses' caring role and the scientific knowledge needed to carry out the role.

As a result of the diverse uses and treatment of the ideas in the book, it is necessary to keep the work alive and available to a new generation of nurse educators, scholars, clinicians and students. The second printing of the book was graciously arranged by the Colorado Associated University Press.

The premises and content of the original book are still applicable; I have not changed my basic views on the caring process in nursing. The ten identified "carative factors" remain the same. However, some dimensions of the overall human care process have been expanded in my recent work entitled Nursing: Human Science and Human Care *(Connecticut: Appleton-Century Crofts, 1985).*

While Nursing: The Philosophy and Science of Caring *was not originally conceived as a theory per se, it indeed provides a theoretical perspective about nursing and caring. Even though my ideas and notions about caring and the human science aspect of nursing keep growing and changing, the "core" con-*

cepts labeled as the carative factors continue to be viewed as intrinsic to the human care process in nursing.

Nursing theory greatly advanced between 1979 and 1985; nevertheless, the human care process continues to need theorizing, researching and practicing. The original core components of caring still provide a structure and order for understanding and studying the basic foundation of nursing.

The human science and art of nursing, the empirics, aesthetics, ethics and intuition of caring are just beginning to be glimpsed by a new generation of nurse scholars, educators, professional clinicians and nurse administrators. Preservation of human care is a critical agenda for nursing and the health care system of today, which has become increasingly technological, medically specialized and depersonalized. It is perhaps the human care process in nursing that helps to facilitate and sustain the person, as an end in and of him or her self in the system, and not as a means to some scientific, biotechnological end. However, the human and caring component of nursing and health care is always threatened and fragile. The profession, the health care system and society must work to preserve the humanity in the system. Human caring in nursing is especially delicate when pressured by the forces of economics, biomedical science and systems management of this era. It is all the more reason for keeping alive a treatise on nursing that highlights caring as the very core and heart of nursing and humanity in the system. The second printing will hopefully serve to maintain and reactivate the philosophical, epistemic, empirical and aesthetic interest in the caring process in nursing.

JEAN WATSON, R.N., Ph.D., F.A.A.N.

I. NURSING AS THE SCIENCE OF CARING

In nursing education and practice, change is the order of the day. The goals of nursing education, the means of fulfilling them, and the bases for evaluating them depend almost exclusively on the goals of nursing practice. Even though educational goals may be as different as the students and teachers themselves, "one recurrent educational goal [that is stated] with some consistency is that of equipping the student with the necessary skills to live effectively and productively in the world of tomorrow" [7].

Nursing education was moved from the confines of the hospital to the university to establish nursing as a discipline and to give the nurse greater knowledge and understanding of human behavior. That foundation helps the nurse in caring for other people. A goal of many nursing programs is the pursuit of self-actualization, as reported in Kramer and Reed's study [10].

The aim of this curriculum is to educate individuals to be self-directive, to be able to think critically, to be able to realize their fullest potential.

The curriculum is designed to facilitate and create a climate for each student to fully pursue her own process of self-actualization and to foster it in others.

Nurse educators must prepare students to practice in conditions of constant change. At the same time nurse educators must emphasize preparation for future practice.

Therefore, the basic requirement for professional nursing is a liberal education, an education that has nothing — and everything — to do with a professional education. The liberal arts are the arts of communication and the arts of using the mind. They are indispensable to further learning, and they

1

should help the student to pursue a lifelong self-education that is liberal and liberating.

The liberal arts are the bases of teaching people to think clearly and thoroughly — the bases of reading, writing, speaking, listening, and valuing [9]. In the past it was held that learning was neutral in regard to values. That view is now being challenged. Educators, especially those in nursing, are again seriously concerned with the full range of human development, including the formation of moral and esthetic values [3].

The liberal arts can give nursing education a timeless quality that is relevant regardless of the changes that occur. The liberal arts are the arts of becoming human and of relating to other people. The liberal arts and the humanities belong to the heart of higher education. They provide analytic skills and self-understanding. Nursing needs to promote and maintain visions, perspectives, and values that allow for creative possibilities. Such a foundation makes the other kinds of scientific and professional knowledge lasting and significant.

In nursing it is easy to fall prey to current trends and fads of education and practice. Nursing is becoming established as an academic discipline that requires a liberal arts education, as well as a scientific and professional education. It is therefore incumbent on the profession and the academic community to adhere to the purpose of a university education — to gain knowledge and understanding [9]. More energy is now expended in the acquisition of scientific knowledge than of understanding. Nursing tries to understand people and how they cope with health and illness.

Nursing covers an area of knowledge somewhere in the biophysical, behavioral, and social sciences and the humanities. It tries to understand how health and illness and human behavior are interrelated. Nursing education rarely concentrates on that level of understanding. In some ways nursing schools are still technical, professional schools. Many teachers and schools state attempts to develop self-actualization. However, they end up hidden, primarily teaching specialized terminology, procedures, scientific principles, the basic content of behavior, pathophysiology, and the disease processes.

Teaching mostly the rules and procedures — the "trim" — of nursing does not lead to understanding people and how they cope with health and illness. Even if all the rules and procedures could be taught (they cannot), many things taught today are outdated in a few years.

The way to understand nursing is to understand it in its context and in its relationship to other subjects. Philosophy, the humanities, history, psychology, physiology, sociology, anthropology, and all the other social sciences affect — and are affected by — nursing. That centrality of nursing makes it a field to be studied in the university. The way to understand nursing is to identify, describe, and research those central humanistic-scientific factors that are essential to effecting positive health change. Those factors are primary mechanisms in "caring for" another human being. They lie somewhere between the sciences and humanities. Nursing today is a discipline that interfaces with the academic world and the professional world.

BALANCING SCIENCE WITH HUMANISM— THE SCIENCE OF CARING

As a university subject, nursing must achieve a delicate balance between scientific knowledge and humanistic practice behaviors. It is therefore important (if not critical) for nursing to realize the need for both a professional education and a liberal arts education.

A conscious effort on the part of the health profession to control disease, prolong life, and alleviate pain has brought dramatic results. However, the humanities and the behavioral sciences address themselves to deeper values of the quality of living and dying, which involve philosophical, ethical, psychosocial, and moral issues. Because of the differences between science and the humanities, it is now possible to define an outcome of scientific activity (e.g., prolongation of life) without referring to its esthetic-humanistic aspect (e.g., the quality of life and death).

SIMILARITIES AND DIFFERENCES BETWEEN SCIENCE AND THE HUMANITIES

There are differences as well as similarities between science and the humanities. It is crucial to know the important functions that science cannot perform for the practice behavior and the important functions that the humanities cannot perform for the knowledge base. Understanding those differences helps the student and practitioner understand why both perspectives are needed in nursing.

Science is concerned with ordering human behavior and producing detachment from individual experiences. Science is neutral in regard to human values. Science is concerned with methods, generalizations, and predictions [11, 12]. However, there are important functions that science cannot perform, perhaps because it asks different kinds of questions than do the humanities.

The humanities address themselves to the understanding and evaluation of human goals and experiences. They are concerned with people's emotional responses to experiences. The humanities look for individual differences and uniqueness. They examine the diversity and quality of human experiences. In the humanities, imagination and insight are validated from within, without justification by scientific criteria.

Because of the important differences between the sciences and the humanities, the educator must be aware of the strengths and weaknesses of each. Science lacks the capacity for humanistic learning because it is not concerned with human goals and values. Science is not concerned with individual experience. Science cannot be expected to keep alive a sense of common humanity [12].

The humanities, on the other hand, cannot give predictable solutions to the problems of human nature. The humanities cannot provide the hard data base that comprises the intellectual content of nursing and the other health sciences.

The new student in nursing, and even the experienced graduate nurse, may struggle with the differences between the sciences and the humanities. Because of their own value systems they may emphasize one domain and ignore the other.

But both domains are important in nursing and the other health sciences. The nurse must understand what each domain can and cannot contribute to nursing.

In spite of the inherent differences between science and the humanities, there exists the capacity for the science of caring that approaches human problems from both directions. The science of caring combines science with the humanities. The science of caring cannot be completely neutral with respect to human values. It cannot remain detached from or indifferent to human emotions — pain, joy, suffering, fear, and anger. At the same time, as its name indicates, the science of caring is guided by scientific knowledge, methods, and predictions. The scientific base of caring integrates the biophysical sciences with the behavioral sciences, and so necessitates a recognition and utilization of the humanities. A science of caring requires the nurse to examine and try to understand the meaning of human actions and values that determine human choice in health and illness.

An understanding of the essential characteristics of sciences and the humanities — the ways in which they are similar and different — gives nursing and the other health professions a better opportunity to complement and enhance the use and applications of both domains.

The nursing profession must identify, describe, and research the interaction of both domains that form the base of the science of caring.

REFERENCES

1. Bronowski, J. The educated man in 1984. *Science* 123:710, 1956.
2. Bronowski, J. *Science and Human Values.* New York: Harper & Row, 1965.
3. Chandler, J. Moral values and liberal learning. *The Wake Forest Magazine* 23:28, 1976.
4. Conant, J. *Modern Science and Modern Man.* New York: Columbia University Press, 1959.
5. Dobzhansky, T. *Genetic Diversity and Human Equality.* New York: Basic Books, 1973.
6. Harcourt, B. (ed.). *Science and the Creative Spirit.* Toronto: University of Toronto Press, 1958.

7. Harvey, O. J. Belief Systems and Education: Some Implications for Change. In J. Crawford (ed.), *The Affective Domain.* Washington, D.C.: Communications Service Corporation, 1970. Pp. 67–91.
8. Hawkins, D. The Creativity of Science. In B. Harcourt (ed.), *Science and the Creative Spirit.* Toronto: University of Toronto Press, 1958. Pp. 130–131.
9. Hutchins, R. Learning the Rules Is No Longer Sufficient. (Remarks delivered in 1974 at the Graduate Studies and Research Center of California State University at Long Beach.) *Rocky Mountain News* May 22, 1977. Pp. 1–2.
10. Kramer, McD., and Reed, J. L. Self-actualization and role conception of baccalaureate degree nurses. *Nursing Research* 21:111, 1972.
11. Morganthau, H. J. *Science: Servant or Master?* New York: New American Library, 1972.
12. Prior, M. E. *Science and the Humanities.* Evanston, Ill.: Northwestern University Press, 1962.
13. Ruf, H. Philosophy and critical reasoning. *Chronicle of Higher Education* May 10, 1976. P. 40.
14. Snow, C. P. *The Two Cultures and the Scientific Revolution.* New York: Cambridge University Press, 1959.

1. CARATIVE FACTORS IN NURSING

The day-to-day practice of professional nursing requires a grounding in a humanistic value system that the nurse continues to cultivate. The humanistic value system must be combined with the scientific knowledge base that guides the nurse's actions. That humanistic-scientific combination underlies the science of caring. In explaining the interaction of humanism and science, this chapter organizes the core of nursing according to carative factors relevant to the science of caring. The term carative is used in contrast to the more common term curative to help the student to differentiate nursing and medicine. The carative factors are the factors that the nurse uses in the delivery of health care to the patient/client. The carative factors are developed from a humanistic philosophy that is central to caring for another human being and that is founded on a steadily growing scientific base.

Whereas *curative* factors aim at *curing* the patient of disease, *carative* factors aim at the *caring process* that helps the person attain (or maintain) health or die a peaceful death.

The carative factors discussed here present nursing care as a deeply human activity. Those factors are not presented as final, because there may be an unlimited number of ways to characterize and produce a therapeutic result in nursing care. The factors discussed here provide a tentative foundation for the science of caring that nursing encompasses. The factors need to be further delineated, expanded, and researched. Nevertheless they are the factors that I think form the whole of nursing.

To discuss the carative factors in more detail, the basic premises relevant to nursing as the science of caring must be set forth. Nursing is concerned with promoting health, preventing illness, caring for the sick, and restoring health. Nursing has traditionally focused on integrating biophysical knowledge with the knowledge of human behavior to promote wellness and to care for the sick. In the present (as in the past), the emphasis is on health promotion rather than on specialized treatment of disease. Because of that focus, nursing is concerned with the knowledge and understanding of "care," which is different from but complementary to the knowledge and understanding of "cure," which is in the domain of medicine [15].

BASIC PREMISES FOR THE SCIENCE OF CARING IN NURSING

The basic premises for a science of caring in nursing are broad and complex ones that provide the foundation for the usefulness of "caring" as a construct in nursing science.

1. Caring (and nursing) has existed in every society. Every society has had some people who have cared for others. A caring attitude is *not* transmitted from generation to generation by genes. It is transmitted by the culture of the profession as a unique way of coping with its environment. Nursing has always held a caring stance in regard to other human beings. That stance has been threatened by a long history of procedure-oriented demands and the development of different levels of nursing. However, the opportunities for nurses to obtain advanced education and engage in higher level analyses of problems and concerns in their education and practice have allowed nursing to combine its humanistic orientation with the relevant science.
2. There is often a discrepancy between theory and practice or between the scientific and artistic aspects of caring, partly because of the disjunction between scientific values and humanistic values.

BASIC ASSUMPTIONS FOR THE SCIENCE OF CARING IN NURSING

The following are the basic assumptions for the science of caring in nursing.

1. Caring can be effectively demonstrated and practiced only interpersonally.

2. Caring consists of carative factors that result in the satisfaction of certain human needs.
3. Effective caring promotes health and individual or family growth.
4. Caring responses accept a person not only as he or she is now but as what he or she may become.
5. A caring environment is one that offers the development of potential while allowing the person to choose the best action for himself or herself at a given point in time.
6. Caring is more "healthogenic" than is curing. The practice of caring integrates biophysical knowledge with knowledge of human behavior to generate or promote health and to provide ministrations to those who are ill. A science of caring is therefore complementary to the science of curing.
7. The practice of caring is central to nursing.

   It is difficult to understand how "caring" helps people to the extent that positive mental, physical, social, or spiritual health changes result. However, if the basic components of the caring process are identified, studied, and researched, they will be seen to comprise a scientific-humanistic basis for nursing interventions.

OVERVIEW OF THE CARATIVE FACTORS
There are 10 primary carative factors that form a structure for studying and understanding nursing as the science of caring. Those carative factors are:

1. The formation of a humanistic-altruistic system of values
2. The instillation of faith-hope
3. The cultivation of sensitivity to one's self and to others
4. The development of a helping-trust relationship
5. The promotion and acceptance of the expression of positive and negative feelings
6. The systematic use of the scientific problem-solving method for decision making
7. The promotion of interpersonal teaching-learning

8. The provision for a supportive, protective, and(or) corrective mental, physical, sociocultural, and spiritual environment
9. Assistance with the gratification of human needs
10. The allowance for existential-phenomenological forces

The first three carative factors interact to establish a philosophical foundation for the science of caring. To a large extent those factors are interdependent; they function together in a process that promotes positive health changes. Since the first three carative factors are so closely interrelated, they are discussed together in this chapter. It is believed that they comprise a unified context because of their philosophical-value laden orientation for care.

The other carative factors are discussed separately — even in separate chapters when the content necessitates an extensive development. Those carative factors, although they are related to values and philosophies, are discussed according to a scientific data base. After the philosophical orientation, the ordering moves from a more basic foundation of absolute values to more scientific factors that are interrelated for nursing education and practice.

FORMATION OF A HUMANISTIC-ALTRUISTIC VALUE SYSTEM

As a given, caring must be grounded on a set of universal human values — kindness, concern, and love of self and others. A humanistic-altruistic value system usually begins early in one's life, and it continues to grow and mature. As one reaches young adulthood, the humanizing of values becomes more established, a point that coincides often with a person's decision to become a nurse.

In such a case, the natural development of humanistic values can be facilitated through the exchange of attitudes and beliefs and of the learning and role modeling that occur between the student nurse and the nursing educator.

The maturing person begins to associate the human meaning of values and how they are related to the achievement of social purposes. Likewise, he or she begins to draw from personal experiences and motives to affirm and promote values [27].

A humanistic-altruistic value system is a qualitative philosophy that guides one's mature life. It is the commitment to and satisfaction of receiving through giving. It involves the capacity to view humanity with love and to appreciate diversity and individuality. Such a value system helps one to tolerate differences and to view others through their own perceptual systems rather than through one's own.

A humanizing of values is derived from one's childhood experiences, including the relationship with one's parents. It is enhanced and expanded from exposure to and the study and exploration of different philosophies, beliefs, and life-styles.

Studying the humanities encourages the freeing of one's thoughts about and perceptions of people from different cultures. A foundation for empathy is laid as one becomes aware and appreciative of different ideas, tastes, and divergent views of life, death, and the world in general.

Past life experiences, as well as study and exploration, help to instill a higher level of feeling, thinking, and behaving toward others. Humanistic values and an altruistic approach to life influence the day-to-day patterns of living.

Caring is based on a guiding force and value system that affect the encounters between the nurse and other persons. Whether or not one is conscious of one's philosophy and values, they affect one's caring behavior. Humanistic values and altruistic behavior can be developed through consciousness raising and a close examination of one's views, beliefs, and values. They can be further developed through (for example) experiences with different cultures, early experiences that have aroused compassion and other emotions, study of the humanities, literary and artistic experiences, value-clarification exercises, and personal growth experiences (e.g., meditation and therapy).

Any one of these and other experiences may help one to recognize and use values to establish a philosophy of life that promotes maturity, satisfaction, and integrity. Altruistic values and behavior bring meaning to one's life through relationships with other people.

Before the nurse can make a social contribution through altruistic service, she or he must resolve some of the problems related to personal and professional identity. While self-awareness and self-examination are necessary for maturing, the nurse must move beyond them and get outside herself or himself to make the most meaningful contribution to self, others, and society. Adler [2] believed that everyone tends to develop *social interest* as he or she outgrows egotism and strives for superiority over self.

Having a humanistic-altruistic value system in nursing does not mean that the nurse must adopt a sacrificial, all-giving, and self-denying behavior. It means that the self should be developed in such a humanizing way that there is an *extension of the sense of self.* I agree with the view of Adler, Allport, and others that a sense of self becomes extended when the welfare of another person, a group enterprise, or some other valued object has a prominent place in one's life [2, 5, 20, 27]. As Allport states:

Maturity advances in proportion as lives are decentered from the clamorous immediacy of the body and of egocenteredness. Self-love is a prominent and inescapable factor in every life, but it need not dominate. Everyone has self-love, but only self-extension is the earmark of maturity [5].

A humanistic-altruistic value system encompasses Allport's concept of maturity. Caring consists of humanistic-altruistic feelings and acts that promote the best professional care and the most mature social contributions. For those reasons, I consider the formation of a humanistic-altruistic value system the first and most basic factor for the science of caring.

INSTILLATION OF FAITH-HOPE

The instillation of faith-hope is the second carative factor. That factor interacts with the formation of a humanistic-altruistic value system to enhance the other carative factors. The nurse and other health professionals must not ignore the important role of faith-hope in the carative as well as the curative processes.

The therapeutic effects of faith-hope have been documented throughout history. Hippocrates thought that the ill person's mind and soul should be inspired before his illness was treated. Aristotle was aware that the theater had a therapeutic effect on the person who became psychologically involved with the performance. Asclepius, the Greek god of medicine, was often pictured with his two daughters — Hygiea, the goddess of health, and Panacea, the goddess of healing. Hygiea guarded health by prescribing self-discipline and a good environment. Panacea used drugs and manipulations to heal [1].

In ancient Egypt, the priest and the physician were the same person. For many centuries Egyptian medicine was closely associated with religion and faith.

Faith-hope traditionally has been important in treatment to relieve the symptoms of illness; medicine itself was secondary to magic, incantations, spells, and prayers. Miracles of faith appear often in the Bible. Other ancient approaches to treatment, such as the Babylonian's astrological approach, were based on supernatural explanations of the causes of and cures for illnesses. Mesmer, who treated illness through suggestion, explained that when he pointed a rod at sick people, animal magnetism flowed from the rod and healed them [17].

The earliest attempts at group psychotherapy used inspirational, authoritative approaches [13]. For example, in 1905, Dr. Joseph H. Pratt held group meetings with tuberculosis patients to instruct them in hygienic practices. Encouragement and inspiration were side-effects of Pratt's approach, and they had a psychotherapeutic effect.

Adler — and later Dreikurs — considered encouragement the central mechanism in teleoanalytic group counseling. Both men thought that success in group counseling depended largely on the counselor's ability to encourage and that failure was usually due to the inability to encourage [2, 13].

In the field of psychotherapy it is established that the therapist plays a critical role [6, 13, 23]. Yalom identified instillation of hope as a curative factor in therapy. Yalom's factor is closely related to the carative factor faith-hope.

Lipkin [17] identified two factors that affect the treatment of every patient: the power of suggestion and the power of the relationship. The effects of hypnosis and placebos, both forms of suggestion, range from relief of minor headache pain to removal of the major symptoms of illness. The power of suggestion (the power of positive feeling) is linked to the instillation of faith-hope.

The nurse must instill in the patient a sense of faith-hope in the nurse and in the treatment. Faith-hope may help the patient to accept information from the nurse and to engage in attitude change and health-seeking behavior. Faith-hope is so basic that it can affect the healing process and the outcome of illness. There is ample documentation of the positive effects of treatments based entirely on faith-hope. The effects of the potent drug atropine can be reversed or even abolished by suggestion. "...drugs and gadgets come and go, how often it is suggestion that produces the cure ..." [1].

Today self-discipline for health is often ignored, and the help of a healing agent — a person, treatment, or drug — is sought.

Many people believe or feel instinctively that illness and death are the results of an evil and invisible destructive force. Many people believe that when everything else fails to cure an illness something still "needs to be done." In many instances the something is having faith in a person, or in a health regimen, or in a belief system to "carry them through."

Some people think that the present era is the "beginning of the end of physical medicine." Medicine is only one of a number of ways of treating illnesses. Millions of people believe that the movements of the stars, if properly interpreted, can reveal their fates. Traditional medicine and treatment are used as adjuncts to other approaches or at best in conjunction with other practices, such as therapeutic massage, acupuncture, and the psychic revelation of one's former lives.

The recent interest in card reading and in astrological and biorhythmical charts indicates that, for many people, faith in the supernatural plays an important role in their health and well-being. The popular interest in Eastern philosophies and practices also attests to the satisfaction that faith-hope and discipline bring many people. Meditation, behavioral therapy, and biofeedback are modern examples of how some people use faith-hope to improve their state of well-being. Such practices are ancient, and they are commonly accepted today. Five or ten years ago they were considered bizarre or not beneficial. Now they are widely used by scientists and lay persons alike.

It is within a scientific framework as well as within a faith-hope—instilling framework that the nurse takes care of others. The interaction within a personal relationship is an important carative factor. Regardless of what scientific regimen is required for the care of a person, the nurse discovers what is meaningful and important for the particular person. The person's beliefs are never disregarded; they are encouraged and respected as significant influences in promoting and maintaining health.

Even when scientific medicine says that nothing can be done for a patient, the nurse can provide care. An important part of that care consists of the various supportive comfort measures and of the timeless ways of instilling faith-hope.

Intelligent people have sought nonscientific treatments of and solutions to their psychological and physical problems. Scientific medicine has traditionally held that those nonscientific approaches cannot cure a patient. However, the current response to that attitude is, "If those approaches have nothing to offer, why do they satisfy and help so many people?"

The nurse who practices the science of caring transcends the limitations and restrictions of a scientific approach because of her or his respect for and knowledge and appreciation of the whole person. The nurse knows from studying human behavior and the behavioral sciences that the use of physical medicine is only one way of responding to the health-illness concerns of another person. Instillation of faith-hope — in one's self and one's competence or in another person — is incorporated into the science of caring. The healing power of belief should never be overlooked. The instillation of faith-hope is difficult to define because it is never a finished process. The nurse must always consider that factor in order to practice the science of caring.

The holistic nature of responding to another person justifies faith-hope as a contributing influence in people's lives.

Faith-hope builds on and draws from a humanistic-altruistic value system to promote holistic professional care and produce positive health. The formation of a humanistic-altruistic value system and the instillation of faith-hope complement each other and further contribute to the third carative factor — the cultivation of sensitivity to one's self and to others.

CULTIVATION OF SENSITIVITY TO SELF AND OTHERS

To be human is to feel. All too often people allow themselves to *think* their thoughts but not to *feel* their feelings. The only way to develop sensitivity to one's self and to others is to recognize and feel feelings — painful ones as well as happy ones.

The development of self and the nurturing of judgment, taste, values, and sensitivity in human relationships evolve from emotional states. The development of feelings is encouraged by the humanities and compassionate life experiences. The recognition and development of feelings lead to self-actualization through self-acceptance and psychological growth.

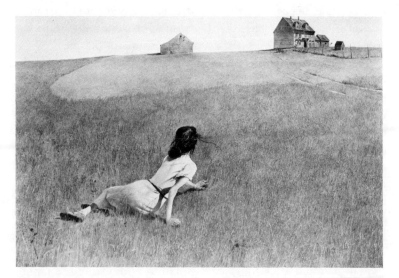

Christina's World, by Andrew Wyeth. (Collection, The Museum of Modern Art, New York)

Most people do not achieve their potential. They tend to look for opportunities outside themselves. But the source for development is within. A starting point is to develop a level of consciousness about one's feelings to look into one's self. People often are afraid to look within because they fear that if they are honest they will see only imperfections. Sensitivity to one's self and one's feelings can be threatening because it may seem that there is no way to handle feelings or that one is not able to change. Therefore it seems easier to push back feelings, to deny them, to refuse to deal with them, or to become consumed by them.

However, a balanced sensitivity to one's feelings gives one a foundation for empathy with others. One must recognize, accept, and be willing to explore one's own feelings. That allows one to recognize and accept the feelings of others, an ability that is related to the fifth carative factor: the promotion and acceptance of the expression of positive and negative feelings. Those who are not sensitive to their own feelings find it difficult to be sensitive to the feelings of others. People who repress their own feelings may be unable to allow others to express or explore their feelings.

Sensitivity to one's self and to others may determine the extent to which the nurse is able to develop self and fully utilize self with others.

The educational and practice situations in nursing often prevent or at best discourage the nurse from being too sensitive to or getting too involved with another's feelings. The nurse may overreact to protect her or his own feelings. As a result, the nurse often forms impersonal, detached professional relationships, in which she or he hides behind a so-called professional character armor [15]. The nurse often deals with her or his own feelings by camouflaging potential conflicts between the nurse and the patient/client. However, the conflicts are not resolved for either the nurse or the other person, as the following example shows.

A young woman had a first child who was stillborn. The woman had had a long and painful labor, and during the labor she had learned that her child was dead. Although the woman had participated actively in the labor, at the moment of her child's birth the woman's face had been covered — ostensibly to prevent her from seeing her dead child. Perhaps the real reason for the covering was to protect the staff from their own anxieties and feelings of inadequacy. The staff lacked sensitivity to themselves and to the woman. They did not offer primary care and prevention. Both scientific knowledge and intuition say that in a situation like the one just described, the feelings of the hospital staff and of the patient should be acknowledged and dealt with. If they are not, both the staff and the patient are deprived of a significant experience. In such a situation, both parties are suffering. If the covering up and denial of the suffering continue, pathology results that can affect the nurse's mental health and practice behaviors and the patient's mental health and behavior. The process that is established in a situation such as the one just described can extend to numerous other situations unless nurses continually observe themselves and their relationships with others. If nurses — helping professionals — fail to be human at sensitive or painful times, they fail at helping. They succeed only in hiding behind their role and their insecurities and anxieties; and they contribute nothing to their own health or the health of others.

The morning after the delivery just described, the young mother asked a student nurse, "Do they always cover your face when you deliver a baby?" That innocent and simple question shows that a lack of sensitivity can make a painful experience even more painful.

Nurses must be genuine to themselves and their feelings. Honesty toward self promotes authenticity and sensitivity toward others, and it lays a foundation for primary prevention. A nurse attains and promotes health and higher level functioning only if she or he forms person-to-person relationships as opposed to manipulative relationships.

Primary preventive care occurs when nurses are committed to high level health and growth for themselves and others. When the carative factor of sensitivity to themselves and others is operating, nurses function as whole persons and can give holistic care. Both the patients and the nurses retain their separate identities.

Authenticity with self and others is the foundation for integrity. From it, an *I-Thou* [8] relationship can result that establishes an empathetic relationship for acceptance, exploration, and growth.

Practicing sensitivity to self and others becomes "something basic" [15] that is common to all types of nursing. Sensitivity to self and others builds on the formation of a humanistic-altruistic value system and the instillation of faith-hope, and it commits the nurse to helping other people achieve such goals as satisfaction, comfort, freedom from pain and suffering, and higher level wellness.

The nurse who is sensitive to feelings is able to make another person feel understood, accepted, and capable of moving toward a more mature level of functioning and growth. The nurse who is sensitive is better able to learn another person's view of the world. The culture, language, belief system, and values influence her or his desire for and concern about comfort, recovery, and wellness. People are always growing and maturing. Health-illness problems and interpersonal relationships are valuable aids to growth and maturity — to developing potentialities as well as actualities. In the context of caring the nurse never assumes that she or he knows the other person, but at each meeting she or he continues to try to get to know the patient/client. That approach requires sensitivity to one's self and to others.

The nurse who recognizes and uses her or his sensitivity and feelings promotes self-development and self-actualization and is able to encourage the same growth in others. Because the carative factor sensitivity to one's self and to others is considered basic to nursing, it may not be explicitly acknowledged, valued, or used. But it cannot be taken for granted, and so it has been discussed in this chapter as a distinct carative factor. Without that factor, nursing care would fail.

REFERENCES
1. Ackerknecht, E. H. *A Short History of Medicine.* New York: Ronald, 1968. P. xvii.
2. Adler, A. *Understanding Human Nature.* Philadelphia: Chilton, 1927.

3. Ainsworth, M. D. S. Object relations, dependency and attachment: A theoretical review of the infant-mother relationship. *Child Development* 40:969, 1969.
4. Ainsworth, M. D. S., and Bell, S. M. Some Contemporary Patterns of Mother-Infant Interaction in the Feeding Situations. In J. A. Ambrose (ed.), *Stimulation in Early Infancy*. London: Academic, 1969.
5. Allport, G. W. *Pattern and Growth in Personality*. New York: Holt, Rinehart and Winston, 1961.
6. Bergin, A. C., and Garfield, S. L. (eds.). *Handbook of Psychotherapy and Behavior Change: An Empirical Analysis*. New York: Wiley, 1971.
7. Bowlby, J., Jr. *Attachment*. Attachment and Loss, vol. 1. New York: Basic Books, 1969.
8. Buber, M. *I and Thou*. New York: Scribner's, 1937.
9. Caplan, G. *Principles of Preventive Psychiatry*. New York: Basic Books, 1964.
10. Dubos, R. J. *Mirage of Health*. New York: Harper & Row, 1959.
11. Engel, G. L. *Psychological Development in Health and Disease*. Philadelphia: Saunders, 1962.
12. Erikson, E. H. *Childhood and Society* (2nd ed.). New York: Norton, 1963.
13. Gazda, G. M. *Basic Approaches to Group Psychotherapy and Group Counseling* (2nd ed.). Springfield, Ill.: Thomas, 1975.
14. Holmes, T. H., and Masuda, M. Life Change and Illness Susceptibility. In B. S. Dohrenwend and B. P. Dohrenwend, *Stressful Life Events*. New York: Wiley, 1974.
15. Jourard, S. M. *The Transparent Self*. Princeton, N.J.: Van Nostrand, 1964.
16. Kübler-Ross, E. *On Death and Dying*. New York: Macmillan, 1969.
17. Lipkin, M. *The Care of Patients*. New York: Oxford University Press, 1975.
18. Mahler, M. S., Pine, F., and Bergman, A. *The Psychological Birth of the Human Infant*. New York: Basic Books, 1975.
19. Maslow, A. H. *Motivation and Personality*. New York: Harper & Bros., 1954.
20. Maslow, A. H. *The Farther Reaches of Human Nature*. New York: Viking, 1976.
21. Newman, M., and Berkowitz, B. *How to Be Your Own Best Friend*. New York: Random House, 1971.
22. Rahe, R. H. The Pathway Between Subjects' Recent Life Changes and Their Near Future Illness Reports. In B. S. Dohrenwend, and B. P. Dohrenwend, *Stressful Life Events*. New York: Wiley, 1974. Pp. 73–86.
23. Rogers, C. R. *Person to Person: The Problem of Being Human*. California: Real People Press, 1967.

24. Schoenberg, B., Carr, A., Peretz, D., and Kutscher, A. (eds.). *Loss and Grief.* New York: Columbia University Press, 1970.
25. Spitz, R. A. *A Genetic Field Theory of Ego Formation: Its Implication for Pathology.* New York: International Universities Press, 1959.
26. Spitz, R. A. *The First Year of Life.* New York: International Universities Press, 1965.
27. White, R. W. *Lives in Progress* (3rd ed.). New York: Holt, Rinehart and Winston, 1975.
28. Yalom, I. D. *The Theory and Practice of Group Psychotherapy* (2nd ed.). New York: Basic Books, 1975.

2. DEVELOPMENT OF A HELPING-TRUST RELATIONSHIP; PROMOTION AND ACCEPTANCE OF THE EXPRESSION OF POSITIVE AND NEGATIVE FEELINGS

A person becomes a person in the encounter with other persons and in no other way [30].

DEVELOPMENT OF A HELPING-TRUST
RELATIONSHIP
The development of a helping-trust relationship depends on the carative factors discussed in Chapter 1. Because the development of a helping-trust relationship is closely related to the promotion and acceptance of the expression of positive and negative feelings, I have combined the discussion of those two factors. The decision is somewhat arbitrary. I could have discussed the factor development of a helping-trust relationship with the factor cultivation of sensitivity to oneself and to others. Obviously all the factors interact for a holistic approach to understanding and studying nursing care. However, the two factors discussed in this chapter are especially important because they go beyond the value system and philosophical foundation of the first three factors and include an empirical scientific research base as a further rationale for the science of caring. There is a steadily growing body of empirical evidence that supports what many have believed intuitively for centuries — that the *quality* of one's relationship with another person is the most significant element in determining helping effectiveness. The three carative factors discussed in Chapter 1 determine the quality of the relationship. However, the development of the relationship is affected by other qualitative characteristics, which are discussed in the following paragraphs.

Nursing as the science of caring must consider seriously the empirical evidence related to the development of a helping-

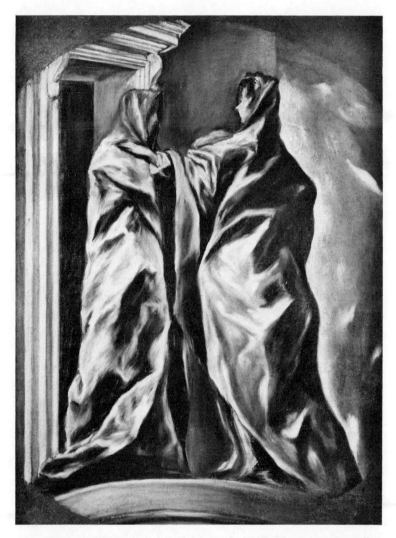

The Visitation, by El Greco. (Courtesy of The Dumbarton Oaks Collection, Washington, D.C.)

trust relationship. The potential for promoting psychological and social growth and development and for facilitating health-seeking behaviors resides in that factor alone if the factor is properly recognized, developed, and utilized by the nurse.

The sensitivity of the nurse in an interpersonal communication encounter is one of the most crucial therapeutic tools for delivering care. Of all the problems that can arise in nursing care, perhaps the most common is failure to establish rapport and a helping-trust relationship with the other person.

A patient/client who feels that the nurse *really cares* about and really sees the person's individual needs and concerns is likely to establish trust, faith, and hope in the nursing care; the person/client is also far more likely to talk about sensitive matters with the nurse who communicates a genuine caring response.

How do nurses know whether their care makes a difference? Nurses who are interpersonally competent are able to produce desirable and valued health outcomes in their transactions with other people. Thus the patients/clients who have had good interpersonal relationships with their nurses show signs of high-quality care.

As nursing research becomes more sophisticated, nursing educators are beginning to devise measures, methods, and research designs that accommodate outcome behaviors, both internal and external, in regard to nurses' education, behavior, and quality of care.

A basic element of high-quality care is the development of a helping-trust relationship. To develop such a relationship, the nurse must first get to know the other person, including the other person's self, life space, and phenomenological view of his or her world. What is the other person's "phenomenal field" that affects, motivates, or inhibits his or her health-seeking behaviors?

The nurse first must view the other person as a separate thinking and feeling human being. Such a view is emphasized because nurses often look on patients as objects of their care (e.g., "Room 303 needs a shot"; "It's time to logroll Mrs. Parsons"). Such an attitude is subtle but pervasive. The nurse must examine how she or he regards other human beings — as objects to be manipulated and treated, or as human beings to be understood?

The inability of nurses to see how they regard other people is so common that it is hardly considered. It becomes an accepted mode of institutionalized behavior. Thus the development of a helping-trust relationship must be acknowledged as a separate and important carative factor that makes a difference in the quality of care.

The American Hospital Association has published a 12-point
"Patients' Bill of Rights" that emphasizes the respect, consideration, care, information, and privacy that people are entitled
to when they become patients. The need to publish such a
document indicates that patients are sometimes not given their
basic rights as people. Health professionals do not intention-
ally disregard the needs and rights of their patients. Often the
problem is that the health professionals lack some of the attributes described by the carative factors, especially the ability
to develop a helping-trust relationship.

What does the steadily growing body of evidence say about
the development of a helping-trust relationship? First the
nurse must bring to the helping-trust relationship certain attitudinal processes. Some of those processes have been mentioned (e.g., sensitivity to self, openness to others, altruism).
Others that have been separated and empirically validated one
by one (even though they are interrelated) are discussed in the
following paragraphs.

Congruence
After years of practice as a counselor and psychotherapist,
Carl Rogers developed the concept of congruence, a basic and
necessary attitudinal process. Congruence was later researched
as a critical variable in helping-trust relationships, and it was
validated empirically. Congruence is closely related to the
carative factor, cultivation of sensitivity to self and to others.
Congruence is based on the nurse's being what she or he seems
to be — genuine and without a "front" or professional "character armor." Congruence involves an openness with the feelings
and attitudes that are within at a given moment. Congruence
can be equated with genuineness. Genuineness refers to being
real, honest, and authentic. "Man's search in helping and in life
is a search for authenticity, both intrapersonal and interpersonal" [24].

Although no one is completely aware of what is going on
within himself or herself, the more sensitive one is to one's
inner self and the more open one is about one's feelings (without denying or fearing them), the higher is one's degree of
congruence.

Certain feelings must be monitored and controlled. It is

inappropriate and not realistic to reveal feelings impulsively. However, the nurse must take on the difficult job of becoming acquainted with the inner experience of self. A nurse who tries to hide from her or his inner self and feelings may use them destructively in a relationship with the other person. Even though her or his actions may be unintentional and protective, they can negatively affect quality care.

Rogers, Carkhuff, Gazda, and others have established guidelines for responding with congruence [2, 4, 5, 9, 22]. The nurse who follows those guidelines will:

1. Minimize playing roles with others, especially the role of the professional helper. The nurse must model genuineness, authenticity, and openness if the other person is to be authentic, genuine, and open.
2. Be able to inquire and learn about the difficulties that she or he experiences with others. That is, the nurse must honestly try to learn the source of the difficulties — whether it originates within or without, or whether it is the result of the interaction of both parties. Doing so may necessitate work with self through counseling, therapy, or other comparable growth efforts. The process is an on-going life experience.
3. Respond to one's own experiences as well as the experiences of the patient. The nurse must be turned into her- or him-self as well as toward others.

The following statement gives an example of an opportunity for a nurse to show honesty:

Patient to Nurse: I'm leaving this hospital. It's terrible. I want better care, and I'll get it elsewhere.

Responses to such a statement could range from no genuineness ("You couldn't mean that") to condescension ("You've had a bad day. We're doing what we can to help you") to a high level of genuineness, authenticity, and congruence ("It bothers me that you're frustrated and feel hurt by your care here. You must feel bad if you think that no one cares. I'll do what I can if you will tell me more about what's bothering you").

Genuineness and congruence are basic to a helping-trust relationship. The nurse who has congruence can move toward a productive working phase because she/he has a realness that transcends the rigidity of role expectations.

To help the nurse further develop and use the concepts of honesty and congruence, I have included a scale that is useful for understanding how genuineness can be evaluated and measured for learning and research purposes (see Table 2-1).

Empathy
Empathy is another essential condition for the development of a helping-trust relationship. Empathy refers to the nurse's ability to experience the other person's private world and feelings and to communicate to the other person some significant degree of that understanding.

Often the first step in communicating helpfully with another person is perceiving what the person is feeling. Everyone has experienced "not helpful" communication — communication that ignored or denied feelings.

Rogers defines empathy as the ability "to sense the client's inner world of private personal meanings as if they were your own, but without ever losing the 'as if' quality" [22]. Empathy has been repeatedly found to be a critical variable for a successful helping relationship [2, 9].

The ability of the nurse to respond to another person's feelings is the foundation for empathy. If the nurse is able to sense her or his own feelings, the nurse and the patient have a common reference point of emotional experience. No one can completely undergo another's experiences, but everyone has felt hurt, angry, sad, guilty, or joyful at one time or another. The feeling states common to all people are reference points that help the nurse develop sensitivity, respect, appreciation, and accuracy in regard to the feelings of others. The ability to sense another's feelings is derived from sensitivity to one's own feeling states.

The nurse who is empathetic recognizes and accepts the other person's feelings without discomfort, fear, anger, or conflict. That kind of understanding and acceptance, which is rare in day-to-day living, makes a difference in helping others.

Table 2-1. Genuineness Scale

1.0	1.5	2.0	2.5	3.0	3.5	4.0
A response in which the nurse attempts to hide her or his own feelings or uses them to punish the person		A response according to some preconceived notion of a role. The response is congruent with the role being assumed but is incongruent with the nurse's true feelings		A controlled expression of feelings that facilitates the development of the relationship. The nurse refrains from expressing feelings that could impede the development of the relationship		A response in which the nurse's verbal and nonverbal messages, whether they are positive or negative, are congruent with how she or he feels. Feelings are communicated in a way that strengthens the relationship

Key: Level 4 = congruent; Level 3 = controlled expression; Level 2 = role-played; Level 1 = not genuine; insincere, phony, potentially destructive.
Source: Gazda, Walters, and Childers [9]. Adapted and used with permission of Allyn & Bacon, Inc.

The nurse who is empathetic can communicate that she or he understands how the other person feels but does not analyze or judge the feeling nor become threatened or intimidated by it. If the nurse is not attentive to feelings, the interaction of the nurse and the patient may focus on facts and thus separate the two.

Effective communication consists of more than verbal cognitive responses; it includes nonverbal behavior and affective (emotional) responses. People receive and give messages through three processes—cognitive, affective, and behavioral. Through the three processes, people connect themselves with others.

The nurse who is responsive to the three processes realizes that it is impossible to not communicate. All behavior — verbal, nonverbal, or action — has a message value. Often the affective and(or) nonverbal communication is the most subtle type, and it requires the most skill from the nurse. Responding to the feelings of another person requires knowledge, insight, and sensitivity. In addition to being the foundation of empathy, which is a recognized helping behavior, a focus of feelings helps the nurse to gain more accurate objective and subjective data from the other person. A focus of feelings also facilitates the development of a trustful, cooperative approach for the evaluation and treatment of health-illness.

In summary, empathy is one of the basic elements necessary for working effectively with others in a helping relationship. It is essentially the ability to tune in to the feelings of another person. Empathetic understanding tells the other person that he or she is important and worthy of the nurse's time. That type of communication brings about a more meaningful relationship.

To help the student and practitioner to evaluate empathy, a scale for measuring empathy is included (see Table 2-2). It may be useful for study and research purposes.

Nonpossessive Warmth

Nonpossessive warmth is an interpersonal condition in a helping relationship that, along with congruence and empathy, promotes growth in another person. An effective nurse is able

Table 2-2. Empathy Scale

1.0	1.5	2.0	2.5	3.0	3.5	4.0
An irrelevant or hurtful response that is not appropriate to the surface feelings of the person. However, when content is communicated accurately, the level of the response may be raised		A response that only partially communicates an awareness of the surface feelings of the person. When content is communicated accurately, the level of the response may be raised. Conversely, when content is communicated inaccurately, the level of the response may be lowered		A response that shows the person that he or she is understood at the level he or she is expressing himself. Surface feelings are accurately reflected. Content is not essential, but when it is included it must be accurate. If it is inaccurate, the level of the response may be lowered		A response that shows the person that he or she is understood beyond his or her level of awareness. Underlying feelings are identified. Content complements the emotion(s) by adding a deeper meaning. If the content is inaccurate, the level of the response may be lowered

Key: Level 4 = underlying feelings, adds meaning; Level 3 = surface feelings reflected; Level 2 = subtracts from meaning; Level 1 = irrelevant; hurtful.
Source: Gazda, Walters, and Childers [9]. Adapted and used with the permission of Allyn & Bacon, Inc.

to "provide a non-threatening, safe, trusting, or secure atmosphere through acceptance, positive regard, love valuing, or *nonpossessive warmth*" [32].

Research on nonpossessive warmth, as well as on congruence and empathy, evolved from the theories of Carl Rogers [21, 22]. Nonpossessive warmth is related to unconditional positive regard, which means the nurse values the other person in a total rather than a conditional way that includes not judging and not evaluating the other person's feelings. Constructive change and growth are more likely to occur in a context of warmth and nonjudgmental acceptance.

Rogers [22] described such warmth and positive regard toward another as "a feeling that is not paternalistic [maternalistic*], nor sentimental, nor superficially social and agreeable." Nonpossessive warmth refers to the degree to which the nurse communicates caring for the other person. Since nursing is viewed in this book as the *science of caring,* such a condition necessary for caring is indispensable for the nurse if an effective outcome is to occur.

Although warmth alone is inadequate for an effective helping relationship, it seems to encourage the development of the other conditions of empathy and genuineness [9]. Warmth is communicated through a wide variety of behaviors (e.g., gestures, posture, tone of voice, touch, and facial expressions). Warmth is an important nonverbal message and attitude that has a positive impact. Warmth can also be expressed verbally; for example, "I can see this is important to you, so it's also important to me."

Some of the important attributes of nonverbal warmth are as follows [9]. (No person can use all the attributes at one time.)

1. Maintenance of eye contact during most of an interaction
2. Use of a moderate volume in speaking
3. Being relaxed and at ease with oneself
4. Facing the other person
5. Having an open posture rather than a closed one

*I added this concept because it is an especially relevant one for nurses.

6. Leaning toward the other person
7. Having a facial expression that is congruent with the other person's emotional state.

The student or practicing nurse may identify other attributes that convey warmth. To further assist the nurse in evaluating nonpossessive warmth, the scale for measuring shown here may be used for study and research (see Table 2-3).

MODES OF EFFECTIVE COMMUNICATION

Within the context of a helping-trust relationship, general principles of communication need to be considered. As mentioned, communication consists of all the cognitive, affective, and behavioral responses used to convey a message to another person. Within such a context there is no such thing as "no communication" or nonbehavior. All behavior has meaning for the person, and all behavior has a message value.

The nurse who wishes to communicate effectively within a helping relationship must be truly responsive to all the modes of behavior that one person uses to affect another. The following are the three basic types of communication that provide a context in which to understand people:

1. The somatic level, which includes the breathing and heart rates, the general physical state, and the related biophysiological states.
2. The action level, which includes all nonverbal behavior, such as body movement, posture, gait, and position.
3. The language level, which refers to words and their meanings. There are two kinds of language communication: (1) *denotative* communication, which refers to the explicit meanings of words and to the overt, manifest context of words and (2) *connotative* communication, which refers to the implicit meaning, associated ideas, feelings, symbolic responses, and latent content of words. Everyone has received or given a communication in which the words were less important than the connotation, which gave the message a special meaning. For example, the word couch

Table 2-3. Warmth Scale

1.0	1.5	2.0	2.5	3.0	3.5	4.0
The nurse has a disapproving facial expression or appears disinterested. She or he turns away or does other tasks while the person is talking		The nurse's expressions and gestures are absent or neutral, and her or his responses sound mechanical or rehearsed		The nurse shows attention and interest clearly. Her or his nonverbal behaviors vary appropriately as person's emotions vary		The nurse is wholly and intensely attentive to the interaction, and the person thus feels complete acceptance and significance. The nurse is physically closer to the person than is the nurse working at Level 3, and she or he makes physical contact with a touch or gestures

Key: Level 4 = intense, nonverbal communication; Level 3 = clear, nonverbal responses; Level 2 = gestures absent or neutral, voice sounds mechanical; Level 1 = visibly disapproving or disinterested.
Source: Gazda, Walters, and Childers [9]. Adapted and used with permission of Allyn & Bacon, Inc.

denotes a piece of furniture on which one can sit or lie. However, the connotation of the word couch may be "formal and not to be sat upon" for one person, and "soft, comfortable, and cozy" for another. Often the connotation of a word, plus the intonation, expression, emphasis, and pitch of voice with which, and context in which it is said, contribute to its complete meaning or message.

Despite the importance of connotative and denotative communication, theorists say that only about 35 percent of communication is language. Thus 65 percent — most of communication — is nonverbal. That fact should not be underestimated in developing a helping-trust relationship. Accuracy in understanding the messages, meanings, and feelings of another is basic to the three core ingredients of a relationship, the ingredients that have been fully developed and researched — congruence, empathy, and nonpossessive warmth.

To communicate effectively in a relationship, the nurse must recognize and value the fact that nonverbal communication is a much more reliable expression of true feelings than is verbal communication. That is true probably because a person has less control over the nonverbal messages, which are delivered unconsciously — often by gestures and other body movements.

In addition to using the principles of communication and of a relationship in a helping role, the nurse must also attempt to understand the *personal* meaning of the behavior and feelings expressed by another person. The nurses' perceptions, interpretations, and meanings may be quite different from the other person's intended message. Thus it is important to validate with the other person that the message/request received is the same as the one sent. If it is not, an incomplete and(or) dysfunctional communication occurs.

To help the nurse understand the message/request of the other person, three basic message/requests are discussed here — those for (1) action, (2) information, and (3) understanding [9]. All three kinds may be given separately, or one message/request may be disguised as another. For example, a verbal message/request for action may include a nonverbal message/

request for understanding and help. The astute nurse listens and looks for all the levels of a message/request value in order to understand the total communication that is intended.

As suggested earlier, the first step in communicating with and relating to another person is to perceive the message/request accurately. If a person's message/request is one for action and the nurse responds by giving information, the person's message/request is not being answered.

A fourth kind of message/request should be mentioned here — the "inappropriate" message/request [3, 9, 31]. The nurse may consider a seductive or flirtatious message/request inappropriate, but if she or he views it in the context of what the message/request might be, the nurse may realize that an inappropriate message/request may be one for some action and(or) understanding. The message/request intended by the inappropriate message/request should be pursued, acknowledged, or redirected by the nurse. A change in the focus of the conversation may direct an inappropriate message/request constructively (see the accompanying model for helping relationships).

Gazda [9] has identified five categories of communication that are inappropriate. They are (1) rumor, (2) gossip, (3) chronic or inordinate griping, (4) inappropriate dependency, and (5) inappropriate activities, such as illegal, unethical, safety-risk, and seductive activities.

In situations in which the communication seems inappropriate, the nurse should evaluate the situation and the subjective meaning of the patient's behavior. The more open, honest, and direct the nurse is, the more constructive the inappropriate message/request can become. An important approach the nurse can use is simple acknowledgment — acknowledging to the person what message/request has been received or how the message was interpreted and trying to pursue the meaning behind the inappropriate message/request. Usually the other person reveals what he or she is trying to say.

The message/request is usually one for action, information, or understanding/involvement. In a nursing practice situation, the word caring can be substituted for the word involvement. Thus most if not all persons the nurse is working with want,

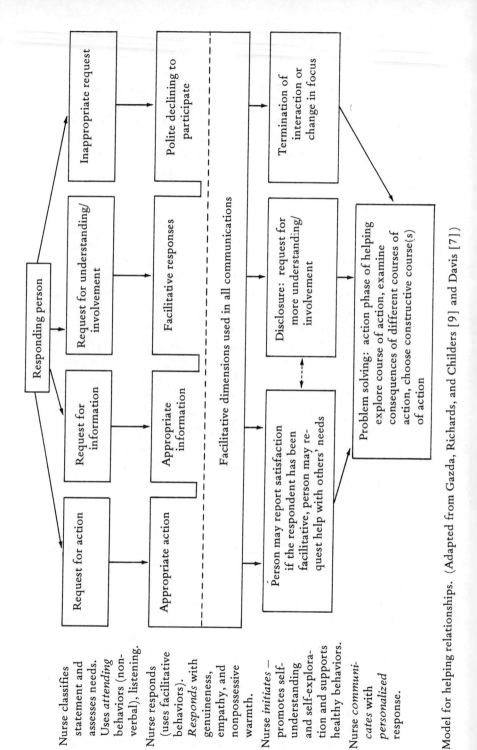

Model for helping relationships. (Adapted from Gazda, Richards, and Childers [9] and Davis [7])

Responding person

Request for action → Request for information → Request for understanding/involvement → Inappropriate request

Appropriate action → Appropriate information → Facilitative responses → Polite declining to participate

Facilitative dimensions used in all communications

Person may report satisfaction if the respondent has been facilitative, person may request help with others' needs ⇄ Disclosure: request for more understanding/involvement

Termination of interaction or change in focus

Problem solving: action phase of helping explore course of action, examine consequences of different courses of action, choose constructive course(s) of action

Nurse classifies statement and assesses needs. Uses *attending* behaviors (nonverbal), listening.

Nurse responds (uses facilitative behaviors). *Responds* with genuineness, empathy, and nonpossessive warmth.

Nurse *initiates* — promotes self-understanding and self-exploration and supports healthy behaviors.

Nurse *communicates* with *personalized* response.

need, and request some kind of understanding and caring.

Other conditions in the nurse and in the other person that block or alter the intent of messages (both sent and received) are preoccupation, emotional blocks, hostility, charisma, past experiences, hidden agendas, inarticulateness, stereotyping, physical environment, mind wandering, defensiveness, relationships, and status [16].

The nurse may use a variety of means to alleviate the conditions that interfere with the communication process. The important job is to become aware of the conditions that interfere with communication and the development of a helping-trust relationship development. Once the nurse is aware, she or he must modify her or his behavior in such a way that messages are clear and mutually understood.

The helping relationship model for relationship development is a useful tool for helping the nurse to be more aware. It can also help in modifying and transforming ordinary behaviors into helping behaviors that facilitate self-exploration, self-understanding, and constructive action for the other person. Those are considered the ultimate goals of a helping relationship.

During an initial helping interaction with another person, the nurse must offer high levels of congruence, empathy, and nonpossessive warmth to facilitate the development of a helping-trust relationship. Those facilitative dimensions further the other person's self-exploration and self-experiencing and thus promote constructive action.

Initially it is necessary that the nurse *attend* to the patient/client. Attending includes attending with the posture and by eye contact as well as psychological attending. It means overcoming any blocks to effective communication (e.g., stereotyping, preoccupation, defensiveness, mind wandering).

Psychological attending includes the use of one's senses, demeanor, and expressions. Such factors as one's tone of voice become important to the meaning of a message.

A voice that we hear, though we do not see the speaker, may sometimes tell us more about him than if we are observing him. It is not the words spoken by the voice that are important, but what it tells us of the speaker. Its tone comes to be more important than what it says. "Speak, in order that I may see you," said Socrates [18].

Listening is an important part of attending that affects the first interaction between people. Listening includes ways of nonverbal communication — tilts of the head, shifts of the body, and gestures. An effective listener asks with the eyes and expressions even when she or he uses no words. Showing that one is listening and wants to hear more of what the speaker is saying is a high compliment and a foundation for trust. In the process of listening the nurse listens for a reason. She or he listens for cues that facilitate further exploration, understanding, and constructive action. Listening includes suspending one's own judgment and resisting distractions and blocks that interfere with communication. The nurse also listens for themes, commonalities, and meanings behind the words that the person says.

Students and practicing nurses can develop skill in listening as well as in attending behaviors by awareness, conscious practice, and examination of their own behavior when communicating.

Often the initial attending behaviors alone can affect the development of the relationship — either positively or negatively. If the nurse effectively *attends* and responds with the three basic conditions of congruence, empathy, and nonpossessive warmth, the other person will be *initiated* into exploring his or her own behavior and courses of action and true *communication* can result, with the person choosing a constructive course of action for health.

The Model for Helping Relationships (see p. 37) shows how the dimensions just discussed are placed in the model for helping relationships.

The understanding and use of the concepts and principles just discussed should foster the development of a helping-trust relationship as a basic carative factor in nursing. The concepts and principles are derived from experiences, observations, convictions, theories, research findings, and conclusions. If those basic skills are not incorporated into the nursing relationship, the result may be potentially harmful, even destructive, for the nurse as well as for the other person.

Developing a helping-trust relationship means that the variable in the process must involve the *person* of the nurse, not simply the nurse in general. It is the *person* variables and personal qualities of the nurse that determine effective implementation of specific communication skills or techniques as well as effective implementation of other procedural technical skills and techniques.

The student nurse and the practicing nurse may learn and use a variety of interviewing techniques and principles. However, without an awareness of the whole context of the relationship, the nurse is a technician or the player of a role, not a person who establishes the trust, faith-hope, and understanding that are necessary to quality health care.

I recommend that to learn more specifics and practice exercises for developing a helping relationship the nurse read *Human Relations Development: A Manual for Health Sciences* [9], a text that was written was to help the health professional develop skill in personal and interpersonal relationships. The book discusses the development of such skill through exercises in listening and communicating in order to problem solve effectively.

I also recommend that for a more extensive view of the research on the interpersonal skills of congruence, empathy, and nonpossessive warmth the nurse read "Research on Certain Therapist Interpersonal Skills in Relation to Process and Outcome," a chapter in *Handbook of Psychotherapy and Behavior Change* [2].

The following quote from that chapter refers to the research that gives validation to the importance of genuineness, empathy, and nonpossessive warmth.

The above studies [50 studies in which control and treatment groups were compared], taken together, support the theoretical view that the level of accurate empathy, nonpossessive warmth, and genuineness are related to constructive change in patients. . . . These findings seem to hold with a wide variety of therapists and counselors, regardless of their training or theoretical orientation, and with a wide variety of clients or patients, including college underachievers, juvenile delinquents, hospitalized schizophrenics, college counselees, mild to severe outpatient neurotics, and the wide variety of hospitalized patients. Further, the evidence suggests that these findings hold in a variety of therapeutic contexts and in both individual and group counseling.

If nursing is to be a science, the scientific basis for the carative factor of development of a helping-trust relationship cannot be overlooked in nursing study, practice, or research.

PROMOTION AND ACCEPTANCE OF THE EXPRESSION OF POSITIVE AND NEGATIVE FEELINGS

The carative factor promotion and acceptance of the expression of positive and negative feelings may not need to be discussed separately since it is an inherent part of the development of a helping-trust relationship. But because it is so basic, it may be taken for granted and not recognized or utilized in the most effective way. Furthermore, there is a justifiable theory and research base that validates the scientific merit of the carative factor for the science of caring. Therefore I have chosen to identify and discuss the topic as a separate carative factor that contributes to the quality of care. The factor will be discussed in a theoretical-research context in the present discussion since it was discussed in a humanistic context in previous sections. The discussion should help the nurse understand the role of affect in relation to cognition and behavior.

Emotions play a central role in people's behavior. Knowledge of psychodynamics and group dynamics helps to explain the power of the emotions.

Research studies indicate that both a rational factor and a *quasi*-rational (affective) factor influence thinking, decision making, and behavior [10, 11]. The emotional (affective) influence in behavior has been labeled "extra-cognitive" [28], "nonrealistic" [16], and "quasi-rational" [10]. The existence of the emotional component has been theoretically acknowledged in the social science and behavioral science literature. Izard [13] maintains that emotions constitute the primary motivational system of human beings. Other theorists emphasize the important role emotions play in organizing motivating and sustaining behaviors [13]. Mowrer states that "emotions play a central role, indeed an indispensable role, in those changes in behavior or performances which are said to represent 'learnings' " [17].

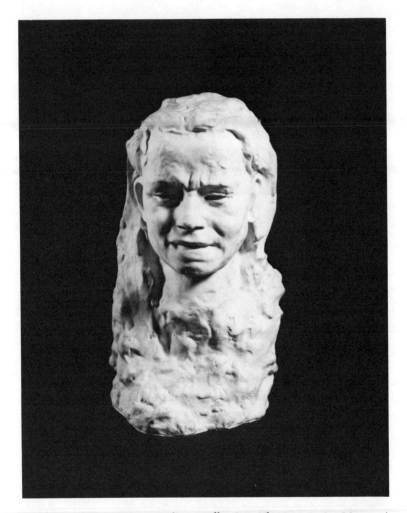

La Pleureuse, by Auguste Rodin. (Collection, The Denver Art Museum)

Social psychologists have used theories of consistency [25], balance [12], and dissonance [8], to describe intrapersonal behavior. Their explanations have usually involved a discussion about the balance between two thoughts that results in certain decisions, behaviors, or an attempt at balance between thoughts and feelings.

It is widely accepted that the intellectual understanding and the emotional understanding of the same information are quite

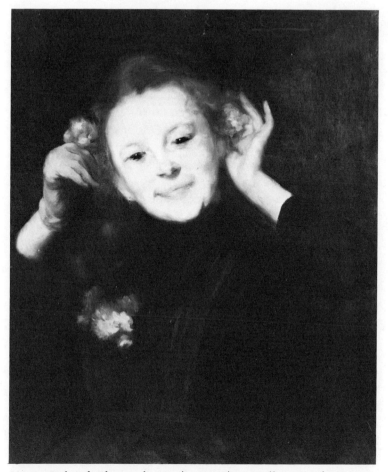

Young Girl with Flowers, by Eugène Carrière. (Collection, The Denver Art Museum)

different. Rosenberg [25, 26] articulated and researched the hypothesis that there may be a disjunction between what a person knows and what he or she feels about the same topic. Affective-cognitive consistency is usually sought by the person. An inconsistency between thoughts and feelings can lead to anxiety, stress, confusion, or even fear. It may alter understanding, influence attitudes, and affect behavior.

In an interpersonal situation, both cognition and affect operate. Cognitions about a topic or health-illness event and the related feelings may explain whether people communicate smoothly, hear each other, listen to each other, and establish rapport-trust with each other.

A focus on one's feelings and the "nonrational" emotional aspect of an event is most appropriate for nurses engaged in caring behaviors. The focus on thoughts and opinions regard ing health-illness matters have been most dealt with in nursing situations, but the focus on affective responses aroused during the process has been often neglected. Feelings alter thoughts and behavior, and they need to be considered and allowed for in a caring relationship.

Everyone has a set of cognitions and feelings that affect his or her behavior. The cognitive component represents the intellectual content. The affective component represents one's feelings about the content, and it is more difficult to understand. The affective component is often inferred from how one reacts toward a specific idea or event. It may be directly expressed in words ("I'm really angry"; "I'm pleased"). The behavioral component consists of action tendencies. It is inferred from what a person does or says he or she will do.

As mentioned, it has been theorized that communication consists of three components: cognitive, affective, and conative (behavioral) components. Social psychologists have used these three components to conceptualize attitude. Various aspects of the components have been developed theoretically, and the components have stimulated much research on attitude. In an attitude context, the components refer to "certain regularities of an individual's feelings, thoughts and predispositions to act toward some aspect of the environment" [30]. All three components are considered important in explaining social interaction. They affect one's view of one's self, of others, and of one's experiences.

Cognition and affect differ in the degree to which they alter behavior. Although the cognitive component of behavior is perhaps easier to explain and understand than the affective components, the affective component is considered a central component for understanding behavior and its meaning.

Feelings are thought to have a powerful effect on behavior and thoughts, with sometimes irrational or impulsive results.

There may be no particular logical or cognitive explanation for certain responses. A person's thoughts and behavior may be guided by certain emotions not entirely within his or her awareness or realm of recognition.

It is theorized (and the theory is supported by psychoanalytic principles) that an awareness of one's feelings may eliminate some of the irrationality of feelings and give one more control over his or her thoughts and behavior. For example, a person may get irritable or angry inappropriately, without even being fully aware of the feeling and how it influences his or her behavior. If the person is made aware of the feeling, he or she may understand what triggered the anger. He or she may accept the feeling as a universal one — common to others in similar situations. That realization may free the person to respond to the feeling with a sense of relief and to respond to the situation in a more appropriate manner.

Even the ancient Greeks made a distinction between cognition and affect. The modern term, *gut level feelings,* suggests that certain basic emotions do not have or need a cognitive explanation. Certain irrational feelings (and possibly irrational thoughts and actions) may not be under a person's control, depending on the person's level of awareness. The science of caring must allow for, promote, and accept the expression of positive and negative feelings in self and others. That focus improves one's level of awareness and internal control over one's behavior and actions.

The affective component of an attitude is said to be that aspect that is emotionally satisfying for a person, a view that suggests that emotions serve a need and that the person seeks to maintain a balance among feelings, thoughts, and behavior.

The literature has established that a change in any one of the three components may cause a change in the other two components. In general, most theories have recognized both the affective and cognitive elements of behavior. Rosenberg [25, 26] in particular has been concerned with the precise relation between the affective and cognitive components. Earlier theorists concentrated on the rational, cognitive causes of attitude change. Indeed, cognition has been demonstrated to change affect [8, 13, 29]. (That finding will be discussed more thoroughly when the carative factor promotion of inter-personal teaching-learning is discussed.)

But in regard to the carative factor that allows for and focuses on feelings, Rosenberg is the only theorist to demonstrate that affect can change cognition. He has established that an attitude can be changed by changing the affective component, which in turn changes the cognitive component.

Rosenberg's central hypothesis is: "The nature and strength of the feelings toward an object or person are correlated with the cognitions associated with the . . . same" [30]. Rosenberg's findings supported a consistency between the affective and cognitive components of an attitude.

Rosenberg's theory and findings have important implications for the science and practice of caring. There is little other empirical, research support concerning the influence that emotions have on human lives although emotions are considered an essential part of human make-up. (However, research on psychotherapy and behavior changes, which are subject to many more complex variables and uncontrolled conditions than was Rosenberg's work, does support that influence.)

Nursing theories and practice are developed around human differences. Individual and group counseling and psychotherapy are based on feelings. Therapeutic intervention and the development of a helping-trust relationship focus on a person's feelings. The acceptance and promotion of the expression of positive and negative feelings has been identified as a major carative factor and a part of nursing's core.

Rosenberg's theory and research attest to the success of an emotional focus. His theory is that certain feelings can change the associated cognition, and his research has demonstrated that effect.

Additional studies support the importance of the expression of feelings [36]. In a clinical study by Yalom, successful patients in group therapy were asked to recall a single critical incident that seemed to be a turning point for them in therapy. The incident most often reported was a patient's sudden expression of strong negative feelings (e.g., hatred or anger). The common characteristics of the critical incident were [36]:

1. The person expressed a strong negative emotion, which was new for him or her.
2. The feared or fantasied catastrophe the patient had associated with the expression of negative feelings did not occur.
3. Reality testing ensued in which the person realized that the feeling expressed was inappropriate in intensity or direction, or that the former avoidance of the expression of feelings was irrational. The person may or may not have gained psychodynamic knowledge of the source of his or her feelings.
4. The person was enabled to interact more freely and to explore more deeply.

In the same study, the critical incident reported almost as often as the former incident also involved strong emotion, but a positive one. The common characteristics of the critical incident were [36]:

1. The person expressed a strong positive emotion, which was unusual for him or her.
2. The feared or fantasied catastrophe did not occur; there was no rejection, deriding, or damage to others by the person's display of positive feelings.
3. The person discovered a previously unknown part of self, which resulted in a new dimension in relationships with others.

Those findings, combined with those of the more rigorously controlled work of Rosenberg, help to validate the importance of allowing others to express negative and positive feelings without feeling defensive and with understanding and support for the expression.

The nurse should be supportive enough to permit such risk taking in self as well as in others. In addition, reality testing can occur for both the nurse and the other person in relation to the appropriateness of the feelings for the situation or the inappropriateness of avoiding certain feelings. In turn the helping relationship will move to a deeper, more honest level that is necessary for the practice of the science of caring.

If feelings can and do change thoughts and influence behavior, the science and practice of caring must be systematically attentive to people's feelings in the maintenance and promotion of health and to people's responses to illness. The theories and research findings just discussed give substantial scientific support to the carative factor acceptance and promotion of the expression of positive and negative feelings, which is part of the science of caring.

REFERENCES

1. Berenson, B. G., and Carkhuff, R. R. (eds.). *Sources of Gain in Counseling and Psychotherapy.* New York: Holt, Rinehart and Winston, 1967.
2. Bergin, A. E., and Garfield, S. L. (eds.). *Handbook of Psychotherapy and Behavior Change: An Empirical Analysis.* New York: Wiley, 1971.
3. Carkhuff, R. R. *Selection and Training.* Helping and Human Relations, vol. 1. New York: Holt, Rinehart and Winston, 1969. Pp. 206–208.
4. Carkhuff, R. R. *Practice and Research.* Helping and Human Relations, vol. 2. New York: Holt, Rinehart and Winston, 1969.
5. Carkhuff, R. R. *The Development of Human Resources in Education and Psychology and Social Change.* Holt, Rinehart and Winston, 1971.
6. Chapman, J. E., and Chapman, H. H. *Behavior and Health Care.* St. Louis: Mosby, 1975.
7. Davis, J. W. Constructive action in the art of helping. *Personnel and Guidance Journal* 54:157, 1975.
8. Festinger, L. *A Theory of Cognitive Dissonance.* New York: Harper & Bros., 1957.
9. Gazda, G., Walters, R. P., and Childers, W. C. *Human Relations Development: A Manual for Health Sciences.* Boston: Allyn & Bacon, 1975.
10. Hammond, K. R. Probalistic functioning and the clinical methods. *Psychological Review* 62:255, 1955.
11. Hammond, K., Todd, F. J., Wilkins, M., and Mitchell, D. Cognitive conflict between persons: Application of the "lens model" paradigms. *Journal of Experimental and Social Psychology* 2:343, 1966.
12. Heider, F. Attitudes and cognitive organization. *Journal of Psychology* 21:107, 1946.
13. Izard, C. E. *Human Emotions.* New York: Plenum, 1977.
14. Janis, I. L., and King, B. T. The influence of role playing on opinion change. *Journal of Abnormal and Social Psychology* 49:211, 1954.

15. Jourard, S. *The Transparent Self.* Princeton, N.J.: Van Nostrand, 1964.
16. Mack, R. W., and Snyder, R. C. The analysis of social conflict – toward an overview and synthesis. *Journal of Conflict Resolution* 00:212, 1957.
17. Mowrer, O. H. *Learning and Behavior.* New York: Wiley, 1960.
18. Pfeiffer, J. W. Conditions Which Hinder Effective Communications. In *1973 Annual Handbook for Group Facilitators.* University Associates, 1973. Pp. 120–123.
19. Redman, B. Remarks delivered in 1975 at the University of Colorado Nurse Practitioner Conference held at the Marriott Hotel in Denver, Colorado.
20. Reik, T. *Listening with the Third Ear.* New York: Pyramid, 1948. P. 136.
21. Rogers, C. R. The interpersonal relationship: The core of guidance. *Harvard Educational Review* 32:416, 1962.
22. Rogers, C. R. The necessary and sufficient conditions of therapeutic personality changes. *Journal of Consulting Psychology* 21:95, 1957.
23. Rogers, C. R., et al. *The Therapeutic Relationship and Its Impact: A Study of Psychotherapy with Schizophrenics.* Madison: The University of Wisconsin Press, 1957.
24. Rogers, C, and Stevens, B. *Person to Person.* Lafayette, Ca.: Real People Press, 1967.
25. Rosenberg, M. J. A structural theory of attitude dynamics. *Public Opinion Quarterly* 24:319, 1960.
26. Rosenberg, M. J. An Analysis of Affective Cognitive Consistency. In C. I. Hovland and M. J. Rosenberg (eds.), *Attitude Organization and Change.* New Haven: Yale University Press, 1960. Pp. 15–65.
27. Rusk, T. N. How to help when the problem is not really physical. *Consultant* 12:59, 1972.
28. Scott, W. A. Rationality and non-rationality of international attitudes. *Journal of Conflict Resolution* 2:8, 1958.
29. Scott, W. A. Attitude change by response reinforcement: Replication and extension. *Sociometry* 2:328, 1959.
30. Secord, P. F., and Backman, C. W. *Social Psychology.* New York: McGraw-Hill, 1964.
31. Tillich, P. *Systematic Theology,* vol. 3. Chicago: The University of Chicago Press, 1963.
32. Travelbee, J. *Interpersonal Aspects of Nursing.* Philadelphia: Davis, 1971.
33. Truax, C. B., and Carhuff, R. R. *Toward Effective Counseling and Psychotherapy: Training and Practice.* Chicago: Aldine, 1967.
34. Truax, C. B., and Mitchell, K. M. Research on Certain Therapist Interpersonal Skills in Relation to Process and Outcome. In A. E. Bergin and S. L. Garfield (eds.), *Handbook of Psychotherapy and Behavior Change.* New York: Wiley, 1971.

35. Vitalo, R. Teaching improved interpersonal functioning as a preferred mode of treatment. *Journal of Clinical Psychology* 27:166, 1971.
36. Yalom, I. D. *The Theory and Practice of Group Psychotherapy* (2nd Ed.). New York: Basic Books, 1975.

3. SYSTEMATIC USE OF THE SCIENTIFIC PROBLEM-SOLVING METHOD FOR DECISION MAKING

Systematic use of the scientific problem-solving method is just as important for the science of caring as is a humanistic approach. One of the biggest problems for nursing has been the lack of a scientific method, lack of quantifying data, and consequent reliance on intuition (or what "seemed right" at the time).

Because the goals and motivation (caring for others) that bring people to nursing are humanistic and expressive, a scientific approach has often been shunned. Even today nursing still fears that an overly intellectual approach or an overemphasis on research will replace actual experiences. Nurses often belittle other health professionals for "not being interested in patient care," but only interested in studying that care.

Generally nurses tend to be too clinically oriented, too work-oriented, and too preoccupied with nursing to address themselves to the larger issues of research, development of a scientific knowledge base, establishment of nursing as a distinct discipline, and confronting bigger problems in the area of national health [4]. For more than 100 years nursing has been preoccupied with defining itself and attempting to categorize various types of nurses (unskilled, technical, and professional). Now nursing is busy differentiating a "nurse practitioner" from a "non—nurse practitioner." Taken to an extreme degree, the preoccupation with levels and labels leads toward the development of a nurse specialist who could provide specialized care only for females between the ages of 16 and 21 in a specific neighborhood in a certain country. Every other type of nurse (for example, nurse educators, theorists, researchers, or generalists) could become a threat, a mystery, an object of distrust, disgust, or indifference [6].

Such an advanced specialist might have a high level of non-personal nursing skills identical to or more advanced than those of a general nursing expert, but he or she could apply the skills in a very narrow range of situations. Persons outside would be a puzzle or a threat to the nurse, and he or she would not want to get to know them. The highly specialized nursing approach tends to emphasize *separation* of the whole into parts. A broader nursing approach emphasizes *connections* between the parts that make up the whole.

The practice of the science of caring in nursing draws on a basic knowledge of the behavioral sciences and on an understanding of how people feel and behave when (1) under stress, (2) well, (3) well but worried, and (4) sick. Professional nursing systematically employs the scientific problem-solving method to help with decision making in all nursing situations. The use of the scientific problem-solving method allows the nurse to draw on common principles and a common data base to problem solve systematically in making decisions and in forming nursing judgments.

Regardless of the area of nursing specialization, the professional nurse has at her or his disposal a knowledge of human behavior, biophysical processes, pathological processes, nursing skills and procedures, and various treatment regimes. The synthesis of all those perspectives and all the data base in the care of a specific person, family, or group actualizes a science of caring. Nursing theory is concerned with the synthesis of knowledge for practice.

Systematic use of the scientific problem-solving method allows nursing and the nurse to practice the science of caring. A systematic problem-solving approach becomes the nurse's valuable tool for "pulling it all together" in the care of a person, family or group, or even a community. It is the focus of the nurse's concentration, and it becomes the focal point for practicing science. Use of the scientific problem-solving method leads to a scientific practice.

One of the biggest difficulties for nursing education and practice is the distinction that is made between the nursing process and the scientific research process. In most instances research and scientific method frighten students and practitioners, although the nursing process is now an established major component of nursing education and practice. However, in the thinking and behavior of nurses there is still a disjunction between the two processes. Nursing process is acceptable; scientific research process is not acceptable — it is something someone else does; it is abstract. It is thought to be not real or concrete and not useful in the clinical work—oriented concentration of most nurses. Why?

THE CONFLICT WITH NURSING'S TRADITIONAL IMAGE

The answer lies partly in the history and tradition of nursing, partly in the orientation of nursing, and partly in the professional conflicts in nursing.

In the past, nurses as a cultural group in U.S. society were "other directed" rather than "inner directed." Nursing was influenced by medical groups, and the professional lives of nurses were directed by physicians. Nurses were dedicated, self-sacrificing, and deferring. They were quiet and submissive to other groups, especially to physicians. They did not question or complain; they accepted. Nurses had difficulty with authority and self-esteem. The nurse was all-giving, and she or he ignored her or his needs before speaking up.

Consistent with those conditions were the philosophy and practice that the nurse learns by doing. The only way students could become nurses was to do certain jobs again and again — "practice makes perfect." The emphasis was totally on practical and applied knowledge. Even though one did not know the principles of a procedure, if one could do it, that was enough. Nurses were very much occupied with the completion of tasks, procedures, charts, physical care, and management of the ward. As persons the nurses were likely to be rigid, conformist, self-controlled, self-regulated, self-composed, and highly professional — to the extent there was no expression of personal feelings and no distinction among nurses as people. The traditional nurse is captured dramatically in the following excerpt from Sylvia Plath's "Tulips," which was written after she was hospitalized.*

*"Tulips" in *Ariel* by Sylvia Plath. Copyright © 1962 by Ted Hughes. By permission of Harper & Row, Publishers, Inc.

The tulips are too excitable, it is winter here.
Look how white everything is, how quiet, how snowed-in.
I am learning peacefulness, lying by myself quietly
As the light lies on these white walls, this bed, these hands.
I am nobody; I have nothing to do with explosions.
I have given my name and my day-clothes up to the nurses
And my history to the anaesthetist and my body to surgeons.
They have propped my head between the pillow and the sheet-cuff.
Like an eye between two white lids that will not shut.
Stupid pupil, it has to take everything in.
The nurses pass and pass, they are no trouble,
They pass the way gulls pass inland in their white caps.
Doing things with their hands, one just the same as another,
So it is impossible to tell how many there are.

My body is a pebble to them, they tend it as water
Tends to the pebbles it must run over, smoothing them gently.
They bring me numbness in their bright needles, they bring me sleep.
Now I have lost myself I am sick of baggage —
My patent leather overnight case like a black pillbox,
My husband and child smiling out of the family photo,
Their smiles catch onto my skin, little smiling hooks.
I have let things slip, a thirty-year-old cargo boat
Stubbornly hanging on to my name and address.
They have swabbed me clear of my loving associations.
Scared and bare on the green plastic-pillowed trolley
I watched my tea-set, my bureaus of linen, my books
Sink out of sight, and the water went over my head.
I am a nun now, I have never been so pure . . .

Perhaps one can get a glimpse of how and why nurses have
detached themselves without even becoming scientific. Nursing's former ethic of "doing" rather than undertaking or learning contributed to its internal professional conflicts as well as
to its limitations in effecting positive outcomes with other
people. For that reason it is emphasized here that science
and human values go together; that learning by doing is enhanced and greatly expanded by learning a knowledge base
and by understanding that both science and human values are
abstractions that guide practice through a similar systematic
process. They both are useful and necessary for clinical nursing practice as well as for nursing research and study. The
student and the practicing nurse should feel not frightened,
threatened, or intimidated by the scientific problem-solving

method but comforted by the validity and reliability it can provide in an otherwise chaotic, highly relativistic, and confusing professional practice.

The nurse must understand that the nursing process and the scientific research process are basically the same. The nurse's learning, understanding, and systematic use of the scientific problem-solving method gives her or him a context for judgments and decisions concerning nursing practice, as well as a foundation for examining the research questions.

How can nurses learn to use the nursing process as the scientific research process? One way is to see both processes in a common framework, to learn and practice them simultaneously, not as separate processes (one concrete and applicable, the other abstract and nonapplicable). They are one and the same as problem-solving processes applicable to nursing study, care, and research. They differ often in (1) the immediate goal (nursing care or nursing research), (2) the extent to which the problem needs a concrete as well as an abstract solution, (3) the degree to which the process is systematized with tangible data that can be generalized from one situation to another, and (4) the degree to which the student or practicing nurse is oriented to them for common purposes and goals.

The ultimate goal of both nursing care and nursing research is the delivery of quality care. The method for delivering quality care — now for a particular patient or in the future for another patient — is the systematic use of the scientific problem-solving method. That method is known to some as the nursing process, to others as the research process. The carative factor systematic use of the scientific problem-solving method is a given for any science or profession, and it is critical to the development and practice of the science of caring. The systematic use of the method allows nurses to collect data from many disciplines and empirical sources in order to develop sound theories and practice parameters.

A PHILOSOPHICAL PERSPECTIVE FOR EMPIRICAL INQUIRY

Without the systematic use of the scientific problem-solving method, effective practice is accidental at best and haphazard or harmful at worst. The scientific problem-solving method is the only method that allows for control and prediction, and that permits self-correction. Without the application of the scientific problem-solving method, the nurse must use other methods, such as (1) *tenacity,* in which one believes something and clings to it, (2) *a priori,* the intuitive method of knowing "before the fact", or (3) the method of *authority,* in which one receives information, opinions, or ideas from an authority and accepts them as laws or givens because an "authority said so" [7].

Without the scientific problem-solving method, one resorts to the substitutes of trial and error, experience, intuition, common sense, faith, custom, or habit [1]. With such methods as those, one lacks a rational, cognitive process that optimizes problem identification, data collection, data analysis, evaluation, and self-correction. The scientific problem-solving method is necessary for the science of caring to study, guide, direct, and research knowledge and practice. It helps the nurse to obtain new knowledge, solve stated problems, make judgments and decisions, develop plans, programs, and procedures, and evaluate, correct, and improve nursing. It can operate on a very large or a very small scale, both of which rely on the scientific problem-solving method for solutions.

It should be emphasized that the use of the scientific problem-solving method often conflicts with the other methods of knowing and it creates a disjunction between the humanistic values and scientific practice demands in nursing. As discussed in the introduction, scientific knowledge should be neutral. But nursing deals with human beings, and so it struggles with neutrality or objectivity. A useful attitude to hold in resolving the conflict between the use of scientific methods and the use of other methods for knowing is to realize that philosophically there are basically different assumptions regarding the nature of reality. Use of the scientific method does not necessarily rule out other domains of knowledge.

Just because the existence of something cannot be validated scientifically does not mean that it does not exist. It may only mean that the scientific method is inadequate or inappropriate for studying or researching the phenomenon in question.

The scientific method does not necessarily rule out other domains of knowledge, it just does not accommodate them according to the philosophical perspective it assumes for empirical inquiry. Its perspective on the nature of reality includes a scientific epistemological rationale about how one goes about knowing; that is, the study or theory of the nature and grounds of knowledge with reference to its limits and validity. The scientific epistemology bases its theories of knowledge on the following criteria for acceptance [7] :

1. *Intersubjective confirmability.* This criterion makes the data objective and makes them public, impersonal, and capable of being reproduced. It allows individuals to view the data from their different perspectives and mutually confirm that the data exist. The criterion rules out premonitions, psychic revelations, and other nonconfirmable phenomena, but that does not necessarily mean the phenomena do not exist, only that they do not fall within the scientific domain; that is, they do not have intersubjective confirmability.
2. *Determinism.* This criterion is based on the assumption that to a certain extent nature behaves in an orderly manner. Therefore, one can seek regularity in the study of the nature of knowledge. Things and events occur with predictability and patterns that can be determined with the scientific method.
3. *Materialism.* This criterion is a practical one that indicates that science can be or is only concerned with measurables. Within the scientific epistemological rationale, nonmatters or nonmeasurables are ascientific, or out of the scientific domain of knowing.

If one were to consider such a phenomenon as the sighting of unidentified flying objects (UFOs) and apply to it scientific criteria, one would discover the following limitations: the person seeing the UFO sees it through his or her own eyes. The sighting often cannot be confirmed by others, and it cannot be reproduced. So far there has been no regularity in the reported sightings of UFOs, and there is nothing tangible,

concrete, or measurable about them. Because of those limitations, the scientific method cannot be applied to UFOs. That
does not mean that persons do not see UFOs; it means that to
date existence of UFOs has not been demonstrated scientifically. It is only within the philosophical perspective and basic
assumptions and criteria for determining the nature of reality
that the scientific method is applicable and valid. Beyond the
philosophical perspective, basic assumptions, and criteria, the
scientific method is inadequate or inappropriate. However, in
nursing, as in other sciences, the best method to date for prediction, control, and self-correction is the scientific method
(because of its restrictions and criteria for validation). At the
same time, because of the relative (as opposed to absolute)
nature of nursing, other domains of knowledge are acknowledged and appreciated, but they cannot be relied on systematically for study, practice, research, or knowledge development.
Other domains can be incorporated into the nurse's knowledge
of human behavior and can be valued as important to one's
self and others. The science of caring systematically uses the
scientific problem-solving method for decision making. It also
draws on different carative factors for effecting positive health
changes and growth. For example, the carative factor formation of a humanistic-altruistic value system and the instillation
of faith-hope may be philosophically different from science at
one level but combine in the science of caring for a holistic
approach to human health needs.

The conflicts within nursing about what perspective guides
nursing have been evident in the history of nursing. In 1933
the New York League of Nursing Education stated that nursing
was "using skillfully scientific methods in adapting prescribed
therapy and preventive treatment to the specific physical and
psychic needs of the individual" [12]. But during the same
era, the essence of nursing was presented as "practical, having
real depths through love, sympathy, knowledge, and culture"
[15]. Those same conflicting themes are partially resolved
today, but they are still present in attempts to combine scientific methods with human values and other methods of knowing.

Because nursing is a profession that serves people, it is based
on incomplete and relative scientific results. Even though it

needs theory and scientific methodology to guide it, it still will not ever be an absolute, pure science such as physics is. The scientific problem-solving method is needed to integrate overlapping areas and incorrect views. Other methods and knowledge domains are needed for holistic care. As Kurt Lewin said [9] :

> The answer is something like this: to make oneself master of the forces of this vast scientific continent one has to fulfill a rather peculiar task. The ultimate goal is to establish a network of highways and super-highways which will have to be adapted to the natural topography of the country and will thus itself be a mirror of its structure and of the position of its resources.
>
> The construction of the highway will be based partly upon assumption, not fully correct. The test drilling and exploring will not always lead to reliable results . . . In other words, to find out what one would like to know one should, in some way or other, already know it.

In order for nursing to be a science of caring in a broad context, it must work within the scientific method but be knowledgeable and open so that it can know in another way what it needs to find out scientifically. That requires the *use* of all domains of knowledge, but confirmation, prediction, and self-correction can only be attained through the scientific method.

To use the scientific problem-solving method systematically, the student and practicing nurse must have additional knowledge for understanding its use. First of all, they must have a conceptual and theoretical understanding of the phenomenon or problem in question, as well as a conceptual and theoretical orientation to nursing.

The use of theory in nursing fulfills three functions that are consistent with use of the scientific method: description, prediction, and explanation [13]. A more holistic view of theory is that a theory "is nothing more than an organization of data, or a way of looking at data to make them meaningful" [3].

Just as the nursing process is based on the scientific research process, the use of the scientific method involves the use of theories. Because nursing is a developing science and has a short history as a scientific, academic discipline (compared to the pure sciences, such as chemistry and physics), nursing theories are not as well defined. However, at the same time,

many nurses are becoming more concerned about the nature
of theory and nursing research and the relevance of theory and
research to practice.

Nursing is becoming more theoretical and less technical,
more scientifically oriented and less based on unrationalized
experiences and intuitions. Today there is a sophisticated
trend toward the development of a body of knowledge to
serve as the foundation for practice. The trend requires theory
and scientific methodology.

Nurses have probably always used theory to guide their
behavior, but their actions were never consciously attributed
to their scientific knowledge. The actions were based largely
on a "simple accumulation of unrationalized experiences" [10].
Today, however, nurses not only articulate the theory (or
theories) that directs their nursing actions but also develop
various "theories of nursing" to establish a base from which
nursing practice can be rationalized.

Even though the student and practicing nurse may not be
directly involved in developing nursing theory, they should be
acquainted with the criteria for a nursing theory. According
to Torres and Yura [16], nursing theory should meet the
following criteria:

1. It should include a set of postulates and definitions of the
   terms involved in the postulates.
2. It should be explicit in its boundaries, its concerns, and its
   limitations.
3. It must be internally consistent, and its concepts must have
   a logical set of interrelationships.
4. It should be congruent with empirical data.
5. It should be capable of generating hypotheses.
6. It must contain generalizations that go beyond the data.
7. It must be verifiable, and it must be stated in such a way
   that it is possible to collect data to prove or disprove it.
8. It must explain past events and predict future ones.

More and more, nursing bases its action on theory that adheres
to such sound criteria. Although nurses still struggle with the
relationship between theory and practice, they more readily

regard theory as a necessity, as a position and framework for hypothesizing and evaluating. Some criteria for evaluating a theory are as follows:

1. Utility. How useful is the theory for generating predictions and presuppositions that can be justified for practice?
2. Choice-Options. In terms of the value system within which nursing operates (scientific and humanistic), how appropriate are the choices that the theory offers?
3. Comprehensiveness. How well does the theory cover areas with which the student, practitioner, and the profession are concerned?
4. Verifiability. Does the theory have the ability to generate hypotheses? Can it be tested and verified?

A theory should be dynamic, not static. No theory is true or false; no theory is sacred or a matter of dogma. It must be capable of being tested and verified. Theory building can extend from the general and abstract to the specific and concrete. That is the deductive method, which proceeds from a theoretical level to an empirical application. Theory can also move from the specific and concrete level to the general and abstract level. That is the inductive method, and it proceeds from empirical or clinical findings to a theoretical explanation.

Whether the theory is inductive or deductive, if the theory is true, it becomes a fact and it is no longer a theory. Because there is often confusion over such terms as fact, theory, proposition, or laws, definitions of the common scientific terms are given in the following paragraphs to clarify different elements of the scientific method.

DEFINITIONS OF COMMON TERMS

A *fact* is the most basic state that verifies the actual existence of an event or phenomenon.

A *proposition* is the statement of a thought that is capable of being tested, believed, or denied. A proposition is usually thought to be true.

A *concept* is a mental picture or a mental image, a word

that symbolizes ideas and meanings and expresses an abstraction. "Weight" is a concept.

A *construct* is a concept that has been invented to suit a special purpose. A construct is a measurable concept that can be observed in relation to other constructs [7]. For example, "ego" is a construct devised to explain a concept of personality.

A *hypothesis* is a conjecture that can be tested, a guiding idea that states the relationship(s) between two or more variables.

A *model* is an idea that explains by using symbolic and physical visualization.

A *paradigm* is a representation of something, a conceptual diagram.

A *variable* is a symbol to which values are assigned, a characteristic, property, trait, or attribute that takes on different values. *A variable is something that varies* [7].

An *independent variable* is a presumed cause of variation, the antecedent of a variation.

A *dependent variable* is the presumed effect, the consequence, the outcome.

An *operational definition* is one that assigns meanings, a definition that specifies the activities or "operations" necessary to measure a construct or a variable.

A *law* is something that happens regularly, a constant.

A *theory* is an exploration of a phenomenon that is based on facts and assumptions; a theory expresses the relationships between facts, generates a hypothesis, and predicts future events and relationships.

TYPES OF RESEARCH IN NURSING
The scientific method and the nursing process overlap for practice and research purposes. They need not be identified, developed, and utilized independently of one another. They both operate from the same philosophical perspective of empirical inquiry, and they both follow a common logic and process. There are two types of formal research: (1) *applied research,* which is action oriented and empirically based, using induction more often and (2) *basic research,* which is more

theory oriented, in which one follows ideas and seeks unknowns using deduction. Both types of research use the scientific method.

Just as there are different types of research, so there are different methods of research:

1. The *formal experimental method,* in which variables are manipulated and controlled. Its use involves a search for a cause and effect relationship that will explain and predict.
2. The *nonexperimental,* or *quasi-experimental,* method, which is concerned with obtaining accurate and meaningful descriptions, discovering facts, and generating hypotheses through such methods as correlational and case study approaches.

Settings also vary in the systematic use of the scientific method in practice and research. There are the following types of settings:

1. The *laboratory* experimental research center, which has a controlled environment.
2. The *natural setting,* which is an uncontrolled environment. A study done in a natural setting is sometimes referred to as field study.
3. The partially *controlled setting,* which uses the scientific method in a natural setting with controls and nonharmful manipulation of variables whenever possible. Most research on people is done in a partially controlled setting.

The systematic use of the scientific method in nursing cuts across many, maybe all, dimensions of practice and research: (1) from applied to basic but mostly applied, (2) from experimental to quasi-experimental or nonexperimental, mostly quasi-experimental or nonexperimental, and (3) in the laboratory, natural and partially controlled settings.

CORRELATIVE RESEARCH PROCESSES
Often the purposes in nursing practice are consistent with purposes for nursing research. Both nursing practice and

research try to solve a problem, make a decision, obtain new knowledge, or evaluate or develop something (such as a program, plan of care, or procedure). Just as nursing practice and research have common goals and purposes, the nursing process and the scientific research process share the same steps. The steps are listed here to show specific commonalities of both processes, as well as where they differ in the specificity or extent of their formal applications.

It is generally accepted that nursing process includes assessing, planning, intervening, and evaluating. Within the process, however, the scientific research process is followed. Study of the 12 major steps of the scientific research process listed here will show that the nursing process consists of the same steps as the scientific research process, perhaps differing from it only in formality and degree.

The scientific research process consists of [1]:

1. Formulating the problem
2. Reviewing and using the literature
3. Formulating a theoretical framework
4. Formulating hypotheses
5. Defining the variables
6. Determining how the variables will be measured
7. Determining the research design or how the problem will be conceptualized
8. Delineating the population or persons to be included
9. Selecting and developing a method for collecting data
10. Formulating a method to analyze and evaluate the data
11. Determining how the results will be interpreted (generalized)
12. Determining a method of communicating the results.

RESEARCH COMPLEMENTS NURSING

The specific steps for the research process can be condensed into the nursing process. That is, the nursing process and the research process try to solve a problem or answer a question. They are methods to help discover the best possible solutions or the most complete answers. The goal of both processes is high-quality health care. The method one uses is sometimes referred to as the research process and other times as the nursing process.

If research methodology and technique are learned and perceived by the nurse as ends in themselves with no bearing on day-to-day practice, a disjunction between theory and practice and between research and patient care will be generated and perpetuated. For that reason the scientific problem-solving method is identified as a process for use in all parts of nursing — direct practice, administration, education, or research. The systematic use of the scientific problem-solving method helps the nurse in finding answers to clinical, theoretical, academic, or institutional problems. The following combined steps compare the overlap and also point out the major differences between the nursing process and the research process.

The Nursing Process and the Research Process

Assessment
  Assessment involves *observation, identification,* and *review* of the *problem; use* of the applicable *knowledge in literature.*

  It includes conceptual knowledge for the *formulation* and *conceptualization* of a *framework* in which to view and assess the problem.

  It also includes the *formulation of hypotheses* about relationships and factors that influence the problem.

  Assessment also includes *defining variables* that will be examined in solving the problem.

Plan
  The plan helps to determine how *variables will be examined* or measured.

  It includes a *conceptual approach* or design for solving problems that is referred to as the nursing care plan.

  It also includes determining what data will be collected and on what person and how the data will be collected.

Intervention
Intervention is direct action and implementation of a plan.

It includes the collection of data.

Evaluation
Evaluation is the method of and process for analyzing data, as well as the examination of the effects of intervention based on the data.

It includes *interpretation* of the *results,* the degree to which a positive outcome occurred, and whether the results can be generalized beyond the situation.

The evaluation of the outcome helps in determining the *method of communicating results,* answers, or solutions obtained — ranging from verbal team communication, patient/client communication, professional colleague communication, and verbal written publication to a more precise formal research monograph. The evaluation of the outcome may *generate additional hypotheses* or questions to be answered, or it may lead to the development of a nursing theory related to the studied phenomenon.

If the nursing process is examined closely, it can be seen that the nursing process follows the research process and that both processes systematically use the scientific problem-solving method. The student or practicing nurse and the nursing researcher need not confuse or separate the two or be threatened by one or the other. Nursing as the science of caring becomes a more complete science and profession as it incorporates systematic use of the scientific problem-solving method. Using that carative factor, nursing can expect and predict positive health outcomes as a result of its efforts, whether the efforts are concerned with education, service, administration, or formal research.

REFERENCES
1. Abdellah, F. G. *Better Patient Care Through Nursing Research.* New York: Macmillan, 1971.

2. Campbell, D. T., and Stanley, J. C. *Experimental and Quasi-experimental Designs for Research.* Chicago: Rand McNally, 1963.
3. Coombs, A. A., and Snygg, D. *Individual Behavior.* New York: Harper & Bros., 1959.
4. Ford, L. Perspectives on Professional Practice. In A. Jacox and C. Norris (eds.), *Organizing for Independent Nursing Practice.* New York: Appleton-Century-Crofts, 1977.
5. Hall, C. S., and Lindner, G. *Theories of Personality* (3rd ed.). New York: Wiley, 1978.
6. Jourard, S. *The Transparent Self.* Princeton, N.J.: Van Nostrand, 1964.
7. Kerlinger, F. *Foundations of Behavioral Research.* New York: Holt, Rinehart and Winston, 1965.
8. Leininger, M. Notes on a conference held in 1968 at the University of Colorado School of Nursing in Denver, Colorado.
9. Lewin, K. Formalization and Progress in Psychology. In D. Cartwright (ed.), *Field Theory and Social Science.* New York: Harper & Bros., 1951. P. 3.
10. Murphy, J. F. (ed.). *Theoretical Issues in Professional Nursing.* New York: Appleton-Century-Crofts, 1971.
11. National League for Nursing, Department of Baccalaureate and Higher Degree Programs. *Faculty-Curriculum Development, Part 3. Conceptual Framework — Its Meaning and Function.* New York: Publication No. 15-1558, 1975.
12. New York League of Nursing Education (Program Committee. Martha R. Smith, Chairman.). A concept of nursing. *American Journal of Nursing* 33:565, 1933.
13. O'Connor, D. J. *An Introduction to the Philosophy of Education.* London: Routledge & Kegal Paul, 1957.
14. Plath, S. "Tulips" in *Ariel* by Sylvia Plath. Copyright © 1962 by Ted Hughes. By permission of Harper & Row, Publishers, Inc.
15. Taylor, E. J. Of what is the nature of nursing? *American Journal of Nursing* 34:473, 1934.
16. Torres, G., and Yura, H. The Meaning and Functions of Concepts and Theories Within Education and Nursing. In *Faculty-Curriculum Development, Part 3. Conceptual Framework — Its Meaning and Function.* New York: National League of Nursing, Department of Baccalaureate and Higher Degree Programs. Publication No. 15-1558, 1975. Pp. 1–8.
17. Treece, E., and Treece, J. W. *Elements of Research in Nursing.* St. Louis: Mosby, 1973.

4. THE PROMOTION OF INTERPERSONAL TEACHING-LEARNING

Interpersonal teaching-learning is a carative factor that includes processes engaged in by both the nurse and the other person. It includes the issues of imparting of information as well as consideration of the nature of learning and what interpersonal processes facilitate learning.

Nursing has always maintained that health teaching is one of its main functions. Often professional nursing has been differentiated from technical nursing on that function alone; the amount and level of teaching done by a nurse who has a baccalaureate or master's degree is expected to be greater than the amount and level of teaching done by a nurse who has a diploma or an associate degree. Patients/clients as well as health professionals expect that.

However, in clinical practice, nurses have often overlooked the interpersonal and learning aspects of the carative factor and concentrated on the teaching aspects. The tutorial method is probably the method most commonly used. Health teaching tends to be done as an isolated event, in which a person is told what to do or what to expect about a specific condition, event, or procedure. The person is told something and given advice or protocols.

If health teaching is emphasized in a clinical setting, it is often formalized into the practice of routinely covering a list of topics and telling the person in general terms what to do about the situation and what to expect. Structured and systematic imparting of information is necessary, of course; many types of treatment are organized today around teaching.

Didactic instruction has often been used to promote a positive health change. Self-help groups, such as Recovery, Inc., and Alcoholics Anonymous, and the Peace Corps training programs and prenatal and child development clinics are organized along didactic lines to facilitate learning and growth.

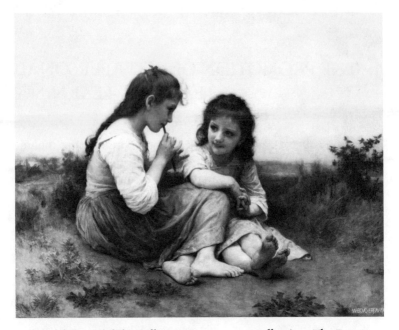

Two Girls, by Adolphe William Bouguereau. (Collection, The Denver Art Museum)

It has been acknowledged in both theory and practice that the imparting of information is an explicit way to reduce fear and anxiety when stress may be related to uncertainty and seriousness of a condition, procedure, operation or treatment. Appley and Trumbull, Lazarus [2, 9, 10], and others have emphasized preparation by giving information to help with adaptation to stress. In that sense stress is thought to occur when a particular plan, sequence, life-style, or pattern of behavior has been interrupted. In health-illness situations, interruptions in one's life-style are most common. The interruptions alone can produce stress, and the stress is compounded by the specific health-illness issues involved.

INFORMATION AND STRESS RESPONSE
Teaching and preparation for health-illness stress have been shown by both formal social-psychological studies and clinical

studies to be valuable because of the many ways in which the role of information in reducing stress may be conceptualized: Those ways include the following generalities about the carative factor promotion of interpersonal teaching-learning:

1. That information promotes accurate expectations and reduces discomforting discrepancies between the degree of stress expected and the degree of stress experienced [3, 6, 8]
2. That information increases the ability to predict what will happen, leading to the feeling of being in control, and reducing associated fears [12, 13]
3. That information fosters the realistic worry and mental rehearsal necessary for emotional acceptance of stress [6, 7]
4. That information changes beliefs and reduces the dreadful fantasies that may be caused by the impending stress [15]
5. That information leads to intellectual understanding that may constitute a method of dealing with the illness and conceptualizing it in a less stressful way [11]
6. That information is intimately involved in the evaluation of situations as threatening and the evaluation of ways of reducing threat [9].

The role of information in emotional response to stress has important implications for theories of nursing. In addition, there are practical implications. Information may reduce emotional response to stressful procedures that are often unavoidable in health care, such as diagnostic examinations, injections, dental procedures, surgery, and treatment procedures. There is a great deal of information that could and should be imparted about threatening stimuli and stressful experiences.

Much data and research are now available to nursing that point to the importance of information in determining and assisting with responses to stress. The data are from such studies as Janis's study of surgery patients [6, 7]; the experiments of Pervin [13] and of Ross, Rodin, and Zimbardo [18] on electrical shock; Lazarus's studies of responses to threatening movies [9], several studies of the psychological preparation of children for surgery [5, 15]; and studies concerned with helping patients to develop expectations about diagnostic and treatment procedures [8].

The science of caring now has data from numerous sources that suggest that accurate information helps reduce the extent to which a threat or potentially stressful stimuli are distressing. Even though there are various methodological difficulties associated with different studies and different research settings, the findings of those studies and studies made in those settings affect nursing and the carative factor the promotion of interpersonal teaching-learning.

Nursing itself needs to do additional research on the importance of teaching-learning to make the data more convincing. But even now the research findings, as well as the primary prevention models, affect health care.

The science of caring draws on and combines two carative factors for primary prevention and health care: the use of the scientific problem-solving method and the promotion of interpersonal teaching-learning. Those two factors are consistent with the problem-solving necessary for individualized nursing care, and they are based on valid theoretical and empirical formulations and findings.

One of the best adaptive responses to stress in general and to health-illness stress is to have accurate information and available alternate responses. In other words, the person needs information as well as control to do something about a situation that interrupts his or her plans and events and thus causes stress.

The nurse must help the other person find "alternate solutions" when undergoing stress. Finding alternate solutions, though basic to nursing practice, must be emphasized because of its importance in interpersonal teaching-learning and the role that it plays in adaptation to stress.

TEACHING-LEARNING BALANCING FACTOR

A useful model for studying and understanding the importance of the promotion of interpersonal teaching-learning to the science of caring is found in the paradigm on page 73.

The paradigm shows (and numerous studies support the

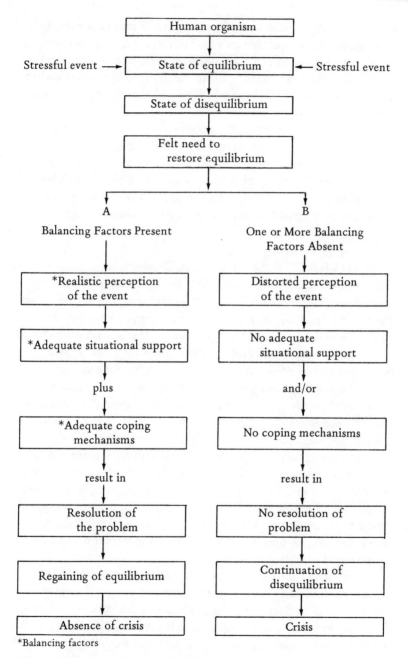

Crisis intervention: theory and methodology. (From Aquilera, Messick, and Farrell [1])

idea) that when a stressful event occurs, certain balancing factors can maintain the person's equilibrium; namely, perception of the event, available situational supports, and coping mechanisms. The carative factor promotion of interpersonal teaching-learning is a key balancing factor and it helps the person who is undergoing stress.

Nurses constantly encounter people who are undergoing stress. Interpersonal teaching-learning, because it gives a person cognitive information and finds alternate solutions for control, is necessary to prevent any further lack of equilibrium for the person and to deal with the present stress (such as hospitalization, diagnostic tests, routine procedure, or surgery).

CARATIVE ATTITUDE AND LEARNING

The importance of giving cognitive information has been discussed here to help the student and practicing nurse understand the validity and importance of the carative factor promotion of interpersonal teaching-learning. Most of the information discussed so far has been related to the teaching aspects (giving cognitive information) rather than to the learning aspects.

As the paradigm on page 73 shows, giving accurate information about an event or an anticipated event gives the patient a realistic perception of the event. However, in the teaching-learning process the nurse must learn what the patient's perceptions are before giving him or her cognitive information. That helps the nurse to work within the patient's framework. Even though nurses know that teaching is important and that it consists of giving cognitive information, they do not always know whether the person learns the information and whether he or she develops an accurate and realistic perception of the anticipated or current event.

One reason that teaching is inadequate or ineffective in nursing is that the focus is on the *teaching* rather than the *interpersonal* and *learning* components of the process. Rarely do a routine checklist of topics and the tutorial method of fact and advice-giving provide any personal meaning of direct benefit to the person for whom the nurse is caring. The nurse must practice the science of caring to consider all components of the carative factor, and relate it to the other carative factors to integrate nursing practice.

Perhaps a more worthy goal than teaching and giving cognitive information is the *facilitation of learning* to improve the accuracy and realism of a person's perceptions about health care concerns.

According to Rogers [17], learning is not dependent on the skills or knowledge of the teacher, curricular planning, the use of audiovisual aids, programmed learning, lectures and presentations, or an abundance of books. Rogers feels that the facilitation of learning depends on certain attitudinal qualities that exist in the personal *relationship* between the teacher and the learner.

If that is true (and there is evidence that it is), the carative factor promotion of interpersonal teaching-learning is related to the carative factor development of a helping-trust relationship. The effectiveness of teaching is also affected by the assessment of the patient's perceptions, which should be made instead of telling the person what to do or to expect. It is also affected by the attitudinal qualities that facilitate learning. They are the same qualities necessary for an effective helping relationship; namely, congruence, empathy, and nonpossessive warmth. Those qualities provide a free, trusting atmosphere for learning and growth. The relationship is a two-way interpersonal process between the teaching nurse and the learning patient. A focus on learning rather than on teaching necessitates a concern for the patient and his or her potential and goals, as well as his or her perceptions of the event or phenomenon. In addition, a focus on learning does not preclude the giving of cognitive information, using teaching skills, and knowledge, or using audiovisual aids and books. A focus on learning provides the proper orientation, atmosphere, attitudinal qualities, and personalized focus that are necessary for learning, which is the ultimate goal of the nurse.

The promotion of interpersonal teaching-learning is a carative factor that is necessary in almost all of a nurse's encounters with other human beings, whether the encounters are specific (e.g., diagnostic procedures, surgery, or medication), or related to ordinary, frequently occurring events that affect health and illness (e.g., birth, marriage, parenting, "growing up," dieting, retiring, care for elderly parents, safety, recovering from illness, or grieving).

SEVEN CLINICAL CARE PHASES

The curative factor can be conceptualized as a form of problem-solving or as a use of the scientific problem-solving method. The participation of both the nurse and the patient are necessary for the interpersonal processes. Both parties can help problem solve. The other person's perceptions and role are necessary for learning. The nurse must be cognizant of her or his interpersonal relationship with the other person as well as of attitudinal qualities and cognitive information.

A model for health care that incorporates principles of teaching and learning as well as of problem solving was recently reported by Pridham, Hansen, and Conrad [14]. Although the model was developed and researched for anticipatory care, it is useful for teaching-learning in general. The model describes seven separate phases in clinical care. Each phase allows for the actions of the clinician to result in specific data, recognizable decisions, and feedback. It was tested on patients, and it has been revised, refined, and tested further. It seems worthwhile to list the phases here since they are consistent with interpersonal teaching-learning [14]:

1. *Scanning.* Scanning discovers problems or goals that are important to the person. Potential as well as actual problems within the other person's framework are discovered, according to his or her own perceptions. The nurse may ask about a range of stresses pertinent to the presenting situation or the specific population group, or the nurse may ask the person to tell about what has been happening or how he or she sees things.
2. *Formulating.* Formulating includes exploring an issue that concerns the person (as detected or recognized verbally or nonverbally in scanning or presented directly by the person), trying to validate it, specifying it, and naming it. A goal may be implied by the formulation of the problem.

The formulation should also include an examination of the significance of the problem to the person. At that phase the nurse should receive feedback from the person (and vice versa) so that she or he understands what is the problem. An astute nurse who is interested in facilitating learning, problem solving, and constructive action knows that often the identified problem is not the *real* problem. A focus on feedback and a congruence of words, gestures, and behavior are necessary.

3. *Appraising.* Appraising includes a joint decision about whether the formulated problem is important enough to work on. At that phase, the available options may be explored to help the patient develop a willingness to problem solve.

4. *Developing a willingness to problem solve.* If willingness to learn, problem solve, or take action is not present, work must be directed toward developing readiness and commitment. That is where the helping relationship and interpersonal processes become critical in facilitating learning and problem solving. They involve the nurse's congruence, empathy, nonpossessive warmth, and commitment to learning and problem solving. It is often at that phase of the teaching—problem-solving process that a disjunction occurs between the nurse-teacher and the patient-learner. Without congruence in the relationship, concurrence on the identified problem, and joint agreement to solve it, no learning or problem solving occurs.

5. *Planning.* Planning involves joint decision-making about how to problem solve, what strategies or techniques will be used, and what the important issues are. At the planning phase, the nurse may be active in suggesting alternatives and knowledgeable about available options.

6. *Implementing.* Implementing includes traditional teaching as one part of intervention, planning, and care. During the implementing phase, giving cognitive information and using books and audiovisual and other devices and methodologies may be useful and appropriate. One pitfall of teaching in regard to nursing care is that it often occurs around an isolated event or *as* an isolated event and not as a process that includes other important aspects of learning.

7. *Evaluating.* Evaluating includes establishing whether or not the preparation or teaching has enabled the person to learn, cope, problem solve, or take constructive action.

The seven phases just described show an interpersonal interactive process that is relevant to teaching-learning, problem solving, and constructive health actions.

A methodology that characterizes teaching-learning as interpersonal problem solving is rarely used; nor is teaching-learning thought to be closely related to the attitudinal qualities necessary for an effective helping relationship. Putting the process of teaching-learning in a primary prevention framework is also a nursing care paradigm that is useful in many health-teaching opportunities.

SUMMARY

This chapter has discussed many ways of promoting interpersonal teaching-learning so that the student nurse and the practicing nurse can better understand how that factor interacts with other carative factors in order to promote holistic health care.

The nurse's role in health care requires that she or he assess what a person needs to know, understand what the perceptions of the person are in relation to the presenting stressor, and the person's need and ability to learn.

A problem-solving approach that includes cognitive, informal, and formal teaching is only part of the carative factor promotion of interpersonal teaching-learning. Affect, perceptions, readiness, personal meaning, behavior, past experiences, and motivation all contribute to the effectiveness of that carative factor.

Because the promotion of interpersonal teaching-learning is so dependent on other kinds of care, it is often overlooked. Modern medicine is so efficient in the cure of diseases partly because it has an absolute, authority-based framework. However, teaching done by advice-giving and emphasizing authority without considering interpersonal learning will fail. That is one of the reasons medicine is so inadequate in the preliminary jobs of preventing disease and teaching people about their health-illness concerns. The science of caring concerns itself theoretically and practically with all the aspects of interpersonal teaching-learning for problem-solving that are necessary for positive health care results. "Without learning there has been no teaching" is a truism that might help the nurse to understand and use the carative factor promotion of interpersonal teaching-learning.

REFERENCES

1. Aguilera, D. C., Messick, J. M., and Farrell, M. S. *Crisis Intervention: Theory and Methodology.* St. Louis: Mosby, 1970.
2. Appley, M. H., and Trumbull, R. *Psychological Stress.* New York: Appleton-Century-Crofts, 1967.
3. Carlsmith, J. M., and Aronson, E. Some hedonic consequences of the confirmation and disconfirmation of expectancies. *Journal of Abnormal and Social Psychology* 66:151, 1963.
4. Coelho, G. V., Hamburg, D. A., Adams, J. E. (eds.). *Coping and Adaptation.* New York: Basic Books, 1974.
5. Jackson, K., Winkley, R., Faust, O. A., et al. Behavior changes indicating emotional trauma in tonsillectomized children. *Pediatrics* 12:23, 1953.
6. Janis, I. *Psychological Stress.* New York: Wiley, 1958.
7. Janis, I. L. *Psychological Stress.* New York: Academic, 1974.
8. Johnson, J. E., and Leventhal, H. Effects of accurate expectations and behavioral instruction on reactions during a noxious medical examination. *Journal of Personality and Social Psychology* 29:710, 1974.
9. Lazarus, R. S. *Psychological Stress and the Coping Process.* New York: McGraw-Hill, 1966.
10. Lazarus, R. S., Averill, J. R., and Opton, E. M., Jr. Toward a cognitive theory of emotion. In M. B. Arnold (ed.), *Feelings and Emotions.* New York: Academic, 1970.
11. Lief, H. I., and Fox, R. C. Training for "detached concern" in medical students. In H. I. Lief et al. (eds.), *The Psychological Basis of Medical Practice.* New York: Harper & Row, 1963.
12. Mandler, B., and Watson, D. L. Anxiety and the interruption of behavior. In C. D. Spielberger (ed.), *Anxiety and Behavior.* New York: Academic, 1966. Pp. 263–290.
13. Pervin, L. A. The need to predict and control under conditions of threat. *Journal of Personality* 31:570, 1963.
14. Pridham, K. F., Hansen, M. F., and Conrad, H. H. Anticipatory care as problem solving in family medicine and nursing. *Journal of Family Practice* 4:1077, 1977.

15. Prugh, D. G., Staub, E., Sand, H. H., et al. A study of the emotional reactions of children and families to hospitalization and illness. *American Journal of Orthopsychiatry* 23:70, 1953.
16. Redman, B. *The Process of Patient Teaching in Nursing* (2nd ed.). St. Louis: Mosby, 1972.
17. Rogers, C. R. The Interpersonal Relationship in the Facilitation of Learning. In S. Stoff and H. Schwartzberg (eds.), *The Human Encounter*. New York: Harper & Row, 1969. Pp. 418–433.
18. Ross, L., Rodin, J., and Zimbardo, P. G. Toward an attribution therapy: The reduction of fear through induced cognitive-emotional misattribution. *Journal of Personality and Social Psychology* 12:279, 1969.
19. Selye, H. *The Stress of Life.* New York: McGraw-Hill, 1956.
20. Toffler, A. (ed.). *Learning for Tomorrow.* New York: Vintage Books (Random House), 1974.
21. de Torney, R. *Strategies for Teaching Nursing.* New York: Wiley, 1971.
22. Vaughan, G. F. Children in hospital. *Lancet* 272:117, 1957.
23. Vernon, D. T. A., Foley, J., Sipowicz, R., and Schulman, J. S. *The Psychological Responses of Children to Hospitalization and Illness.* Springfield, Ill.: Thomas, 1965.

5. PROVISION FOR A SUPPORTIVE, PROTECTIVE, AND(OR) CORRECTIVE MENTAL, PHYSICAL, SOCIOCULTURAL, AND SPIRITUAL ENVIRONMENT

A number of variables affect a person's life and well-being; those same variables should be considered in day-to-day nursing care. They are the routine functions and activities of the nurse that promote or restore health, prevent illness, or care for the sick. Those functions are discussed together as one major carative factor: provision for a supportive, protective and(or) corrective mental, physical, sociocultural, and spiritual environment. (For simplicity, that factor will be referred to in this chapter as carative factor No. 8.) Some of the variables are functions external to the person. They are physical or social environmental activities and manipulations that the nurse uses to provide support, protection, and safety for the other person. Other variables in carative factor No. 8 are functions that are internal to a person. They are supportive, protective, and(or) corrective activities that the nurse provides for a person's mental, spiritual, and sociocultural harmony and well-being.

Carative factor No. 8 does not include everything, but it helps the student nurse and the practicing nurse to conceptualize a major part of what nursing care is from the perspective of the science of caring.

The interdependence of external and internal environments is known to influence strongly health and illness. Internal biological and physiological regulatory mechanisms support the pattern of one's life-style. Likewise, one's external life-style contributes to his or her internal homeostasis. Epidemiological studies have shown that housing, nutrition, income, occupation, education, and sanitation are more important health variables than increasing the number of hospitals, clinics, health-care workers, and cures for disease.

Internal regulatory mechanisms, such as mental and spiritual well-being and sociocultural beliefs, are also critically important to the health of persons. The nurse should provide support, protection, or correction for the various components of the internal environment — biophysical, mental, spiritual, and sociocultural. The mental, spiritual, and sociocultural components of the internal environment are discussed in the following paragraphs. (The biophysical part is discussed in the section on human needs, but not to a great extent because the biophysical needs are considered to be a given and known focus of nursing care. The reader is referred to other, more complete specialized texts to find information on the biophysical aspects of care. The other major components of the carative factor are discussed in terms consistent with the other carative factors.)

In addition to the external variables identified in broad epidemiological studies, other variables affect the external environment with which the nurse often deals. The external environment includes such factors as stress-change, comfort, privacy, safety, and clean-esthetic surroundings.

EXTERNAL VARIABLES

Stress-change results from and includes anything that interrupts one's usual, planned activities. Stress is magnified according to the person's instantaneous and intuitive appraisal of the interruption and whether the situation arouses an anticipation of harm-threat or of challenge. The interruption changes inherent in health-illness conditions endanger a person's psychological and physical organization [1, 12]. A changed health maintenance regimen, as well as an illness, can upset one's usual activities, as could a move from (1) one house to another, (2) one job to another, (3) a change of status to being married, divorced, or widowed, (4) a wife or husband to a wife and mother or a husband and father role. Any such change in one's external environment creates stress, and it requires coping. Any such change may arouse an anticipation of harm-threat or challenge, or it may endanger one's previously established psychological organization.

One of the first most appropriate activities for the nurse related to stress-change is to obtain the patient's subjective, instantaneous, and intuitive appraisal of the stress-change. The intuitive, subjective appraisal creates distortions and inaccurate perceptions that lead to fear, anxiety, and anticipation of harm. Once the nurse has the subjective data she or he can reduce the patient's anxiety by listening, accepting, and understanding. By first obtaining the subjective data, the nurse can better understand the person's concerns about and distortions of the situation. Later the nurse can proceed to the objective nature of the stress-change and help the person to develop a more realistic and accurate perception of the situation. Not only does the person thus gain accuracy of perception but also the cognitive information given by the nurse strengthens the person's coping mechanisms. If psychological resources are needed, the person becomes prepared after gaining structured expectations of the threatening event. The nurse at that point becomes helpful by providing herself or himself as a situational support or assuring that situational supports are available to the person (e.g., family, health team, and community agencies).

Through the process of obtaining subjective data from the person and providing objective data, the person can be assisted with basic coping and directly or indirectly provided with situational supports.

The nurse further intervenes with appraisal of the stress-change by the health maintenance role, which involves the carative factors previously discussed as well as supportive activities. Under stress-change, the supportive, protective and(or) corrective nursing activities are (1) a humanistic orientation to the person, (2) the ability to instill faith-hope, (3) sensitivity to one's self and to the other person, (4) development of a helping-trust relationship, (5) promotion and acceptance of the expression of positive and negative feelings, (6) systematic use of the scientific problem-solving method, and (7) the promotion of interpersonal teaching-learning.

Activities Nos. 1 to 3 are more *supportive* for the person, whereas activities Nos. 4 and 5 are potentially *supportive, protective,* and *corrective* for the person in a primary prevention

sense. Activities Nos. 6 and 7 contribute to the potential of
all three components of the carative factor, namely, support,
protection, and correction.

A TOOL FOR QUANTIFYING CHANGE

The findings of research on stress-change seem to validate some
remarkable correlations between the occurrence of illness and
change (for better or worse) in one's life-style [9, 25]. Such
tools as the Social Readjustment Rating Scale (see Table 5-1)
help one to direct his or her activities with oneself and others
related to external stress-change.

The Social Readjustment Rating Scale is a table that assigns
points to common changes. When enough changes occur in
one year to add up to 150 points, the collective changes are
described as a mild life change. A score of 200 to 300 points
indicates a moderate life change, and one of more than 300
points indicates a major life change.

A method called psychophysics [26] was used to construct
the Social Readjustment Rating Scale. The scale lists 43 life-
event items that require change in individual adjustment (e.g.,
death of spouse, divorce, marriage, personal injury, retirement
from work, being fired, sexual difficulties, major change in
family's health, and addition of a new family member). The
changes are both positive and negative; they can be for better or
for worse, depending on a person's perception and awareness of
the change issue, coping mechanisms, and situational supports.

Table 5-1 gives a list of the life changes and the rank and mean
value of each one. The nurse can use the scale to assess the
person's degree of stress-change and guide the direction for
primary, secondary, or tertiary prevention and care.

There is much clinical evidence to support the proposition
that the greater the life change, the greater the probability that
the life change will be associated with disease onset and the
greater the probability that the population at risk will experience diseases [8, 18, 25].

There is also a strong correlation between the magnitude of
the life change and the seriousness of the illness experienced.
Major health changes that have been observed to be related to

Table 5-1. Social Readjustment Rating Scale

Rank	Life Event	Mean Value
1	Death of spouse	100
2	Divorce	73
3	Marital separation	65
4	Jail term	63
5	Death of close family member	63
6	Personal injury or illness	53
7	Marriage	50
8	Fired at work	47
9	Marital reconciliation	45
10	Retirement	45
11	Change in health of family member	44
12	Pregnancy	40
13	Sex difficulties	39
14	Gain of new family member	39
15	Business readjustment	39
16	Change in financial state	38
17	Death of close friend	37
18	Change to different line of work	36
19	Change in number of arguments with spouse	35
20	Mortgage over $10,000	31
21	Foreclosure of mortgage or loan	30
22	Change in responsibilities at work	29
23	Son or daughter leaving home	29
24	Trouble with in-laws	29
25	Outstanding personal achievement	28
26	Spouse begin or stop work	26
27	Begin or end school	26
28	Change in living conditions	25
29	Revision of personal habits	24
30	Trouble with boss	23
31	Change in work hours or conditions	20
32	Change in residence	20
33	Change in schools	20
34	Change in recreation	19
35	Change in church activities	19
36	Change in social activities	18
37	Mortgage or loan less than $10,000	17
38	Change in sleeping habits	16
39	Change in number of family get-togethers	15
40	Change in eating habits	15
41	Vacation	13
42	Christmas	12
43	Minor violations of the law	11

Mild life crisis: 150 points; moderate life crisis: 200 to 300 points; major life crisis: 300 points or more.

life change cover a wide range of psychiatric, medical, and surgical diseases [19, 28, 30]. Such clinical evidence has profound and valuable implications for guiding nursing as the science of caring. The scientific evidence for nursing practice, study, and research is related to such clinical evidence as is reported here on life changes. It is also related to nursing's role in preventing the onset of illness and intervening with a life change.

The following propositions and conclusions are based on scientific, clinical evidence that helps the nurse actualize the carative factor No. 8 as related to stress-change. Those conclusions help the nurse discriminate in the application of the clinical evidence. They are based on holistic ideas of change, including cultural change, social change, and changes in interpersonal relationships. The scientific propositions are [6]:

1. Exposure to cultural change, social change, and changes in interpersonal relationships may cause a significant change in health if (a) the person has already an illness or a susceptibility to illness and perceives the change as important, (b) there is a significant change in the person's activities, habits, diet, exposure to disease-causing agents, or the physical characteristics of the environment.
2. Exposure to cultural change, social change, and changes in interpersonal relationships may cause no significant change in health if (a) the person has no illness or susceptibility to illness or if he or she does not perceive the change as important and (b) there is no significant change in the person's activities, habits, diet, exposure to disease-causing agents, or the physical characteristics of the environment.

Those two broad conclusions emphasize the need to determine how a person perceives the change, the degree of importance he or she places on it, and how the change affects other aspects of the person's life. A change causes stress only because of the meaning it has for the person experiencing it. Thus the nurse must use and integrate several carative factors to respond accurately to the person's health needs. Routine use of the Social Readjustment Rating Scale without assessing the subjective importance of changes for the person involved is ineffective. Nevertheless, such a device can be highly effective for giving direction and a scientific rationale for nursing care related to provision of a supportive, protective, and(or) corrective environment for stress-change condition.

Assessment of the objective stress-change (using a device like the Social Readjustment Rating Scale in conjunction with the personalized subjective data) provides the following kinds of direction for nursing plans and intervention strategies: (1) giving anticipatory guidance in regard to an upcoming change, (2) giving objective cognitive information to promote accurate, realistic perceptions, (3) structuring another person's expectations of threatening events, (4) supporting existent coping mechanisms, (5) engaging the other person in a helping relationship for constructive problem solving, and (6) assuring situational supports.

It was found from prognosis studies of patients with medical illnesses that long-term prognoses were more accurate when the health professional took into account the patient's social stresses [7, 24]. The predicting team considered not only the occurrence of a potentially stressful situation in the life of each person treated but also whether the situation was producing distress, that is, whether the stress was too great for the person's adaptive capacities or whether he or she had adequate coping mechanisms and situational supports. The prognosis assessment included the appropriate information for future prevention as well as immediate intervention needs.

The nurse should not only attempt to see correlations between potentially stressful events and symptoms but also to learn the significance of those events for the person. In addition, the person's accuracy of understanding and perception of the events should be assessed, and his or her coping mechanisms and situational supports should be evaluated. Reliance on carative factors for intervention can help the person not only with his or her immediate environment but also with future events and possibly prevent the onset of disease or make better prognoses possible.

Nursing intervention can be supportive and can protect the patient from unnecessary stress or correct his or her distortion and faulty problem-solving approaches of the past. Nursing evaluation and outcome research related to life change and nursing interventions would be appropriate and valuable to the scientific community as well as in regard to health care for the future. Consideration of carative factor No. 8 as well as others that relate to stress-change is an important part of health care and the onset of illness. There is now a baseline of clinical evidence about stress-change that nursing must examine in order to develop the science of caring.

COMFORT

Comfort is an external variable that the nurse can control, because comfort can come from the external environment that is controlled in part by the nurse. Comfort activities can be supportive, protective, or even corrective for a person's internal and external environments. At the same time, the nurse's way of comforting should help the person to function as effectively and efficiently as the limits of his or her health-illness status permit. Comfort that is limited mainly to conserving the patient's energy may not promote good health. An oversolicitous nurse can foster unhealthy dependency. At the same time, comfort and its importance for the health and care of the sick are basic parts of nursing intervention.

The properties of a patient's environment become essential considerations for the nurse who comforts the patient. Because of the stress that hospitalization causes, the properties of a patient's hospital environment become critical for his or her mental and physical well-being.

Often the loss of one's identity and loss of independence that are associated with hospitalization are compounded by the care given by a procedure oriented staff that has difficulty in achieving meaningful interpersonal relationships. When that is so, it becomes important that the nurse give comfort through carative factor No. 8.

In spite of many changes in recent years, the physical environment in hospitals is still too inflexible and bound by tradition to meet the individual needs of the patients. Hospital rooms are set up for the convenience of the hospital's staff.

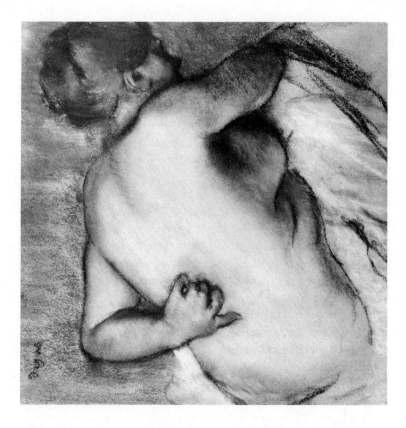

Femme Se Grattant, by Edgar Hilaire Degas. (Collection, The Denver Art Museum)

The wall units for suction, oxygen, and so on are obstacles to room arrangements in spite of their usefulness.

The patient learns on entering a hospital to delegate as much responsibility as possible to the staff. For that reason the nurse must be especially aware of the depersonalized features of the hospital and she or he must provide the most supportive, protective, or corrective environment possible.

The nurse can use many procedural-fundamental nursing measures to provide and promote physical comfort; for example, "morning, afternoon, and evening care," the Sitz bath, mouth care, bedmaking, and the administration of medication.

Other, more comprehensive, comfort measures the nurse can take to provide a supportive, protective, or corrective environment are as follows [2]:

1. Removing noxious stimuli from the external environment (e.g., bright lights, loud or sudden noises, inadequate heating and ventilation, and untidy surroundings).
2. Giving attention to the position of the patient and frequently changing her or his position.
3. Making the bed comfortable.
4. Relieving muscle tension by range-of-motion exercises, a back rub, or a therapeutic massage.
5. Performing therapeutic procedures (e.g., applying warm, moist packs, giving a warm bath, administering prescribed pain-relieving medications, inhalation exercises, and treatment, relaxation, and meditation exercises).
6. Identifying the implications of illness for the patient and the use of the available resources for support or protection. Preparing the patient for what to expect and what is expected while maximizing the patient's control, choices, and alternatives.
7. Modifying approaches to the patient in relation to the severity, extent, and phase of care.

In addition to the more procedural measures, the nurse should use openness, awareness, flexibility, and creativity to determine and develop appropriate supportive, protective, or corrective actions for each patient. A variety of things may provide comfort for a patient; for example, proper placement of the bed in the room, giving a bed bath, sitting by the bed, and contacting the patient's family. Some comfort measures may be environmental; for example, rearranging the room and closing or opening the window. Others may be physical; for example, giving mouth care and a back rub, changing body position, and changing the bed linens. Still other measures may provide mental comfort; for example, listening to the patient talk about his or her fears, helping the patient understand what to expect, and reducing noise so that the patient can rest.

Sociocultural comfort measures should be related to the normal behaviors and habitual ways of the patient's culture, family life, or social class. One's *culture* consists of all the learned ways of doing, feeling, and thinking that are transmitted from one generation to the next (e.g., knowledge, skills, art, morals, law, customs, and habits) [22]. One receives shared assumptions, attitudes, roles, and values from one's sociocultural and family experiences. One's *social class* is a cultural grouping of persons with similar status (in regard to economics, age, sex, personal endowments, and so on), lifestyle, values, ideas, interests, attitudes, and overt forms of behavior [5, 22]. One's culture, subculture, social class, and family life provide values that determine how one should behave in various situations and what goals one should pursue and how.

Furthermore these important variables dictate one's reactions to threat and stress-change, and they determine what comfort measures should be taken. The nurse must consider the patient's sociocultural values, beliefs, and background in planning and providing comfort measures. Carative factor No. 8 is ineffective in all aspects of support, protection, or correction if the assessment, plan, intervention, and evaluation are not accommodated to the sociocultural environment. Because sociocultural influences are complex and pervasive, the supportive, protective, and corrective environment the nurse provides is variable and highly dependent on the patient. Interventions may range from making certain foods available, following dietary taboos, and using special methods for hygiene to considering adjunctive treatment or interventions that differ from, but add to, traditional scientific medical and nursing practices.

An example of a supportive comfort measure that is related to sociocultural beliefs is provided by the Mende tribe of Sierra Leone [14]. In that tribe, healing practices include application of herbs to the part of the body that hurts. The only medicine that is taken internally is an herbal tea for colds or fevers; all other medication is applied locally and externally.

Whenever the Mende became acquainted with the white man's medicine for headaches — aspirin — they would request it for

their headaches. Even though they were told to take it internally, they ground up the aspirin and applied it to the part of
the head that hurt.

Even though the situation is uncommon, an analogy can be
drawn. The sociocultural belief of the person must be considered in providing comfort. Comfort (and relief of discomfort) is highly dependent on internal as well as sociocultural
perceptions about one's health and how to improve it.

Some recent findings of pain research indicate that a person
may report the presence of "no pain" but the highest degree
of discomfort [11]. Within that context, comfort is related
to complex internal and external mechanisms. Likewise, nursing comfort measures must be highly responsive to the mental,
sociocultural, physical, and even spiritual environment of the
person.

The nurse's acknowledgment, appreciation, and respect for
the spiritual meaning in a person's life (regardless of how unusual the person's belief is) can be comforting to the person.
Spiritual and religious awareness is one of the nurse's responsibilities. Nurses now have an opportunity, as well as an obligation, to become familiar with the religious and spiritual
influences in a person's life. World religions, not just a country's religion, are now major organizing components of life.

The comfort measures that the nurse attempts to provide
through carative factor No. 8 use a knowledge and understanding of basic beliefs, dietary laws, ideas about health and
illness, the body, the spirit, mysticism, pragmatism, pain, death,
cleanliness, and family ties. The comfort that the nurse provides in the spiritual realm is related to the spiritual appreciation and respect that allows the nurse to be a link between the
person and her or his spiritual needs.

A team approach to holistic caring incorporates spirituality
as an integral part of a person's needs and concerns. A chap-
lain (or another spiritual leader) may be a member of the
hospital staff. In addition, the nurse can keep a list of spiritual
leaders to contact whenever necessary [22].

Providing a suitable environment for a spiritual session is a
responsibility the nurse can pursue; for example, by arranging
for privacy, candles, an out-of-doors setting, flowers, or a

personalized, nonsterile environment. Any of those environmental measures or others that are appropriate for the situation and person are conducive to comfort and the relief of
mental anguish. The student nurse and the practicing nurse
are referred to *Nursing Concepts for Health Promotion* [22] ,
which summarizes information about the major religions.
Environmental comfort measures are essential for nursing
study, practice, and research. Knowledge of them is helpful
in day-to-day practice and study related to spirituality.

PRIVACY

Privacy is a major factor to consider with carative factor No. 8.
The depersonalization that occurs with hospitalization and the
intimate questions, procedures, and treatments connected with
hospitalization contribute to the privacy concerns of the person. The expectation of the hospital staff that the patient will
share intimate information and expose his or her body without
reserve also contributes to the patient's loss of privacy. Often
the basic support, protection, or correction that the nurse provides in the patient's external environment is intended to preserve the patient's privacy.

Privacy has been linked to health. Maslow's early findings
showed that healthy subjects have a very strong liking for privacy, even a need for it [17] .

Privacy concerns have been interpreted to include [3] :

1. The right to exclude others from certain knowledge about
   one's self.
2. The awareness and appreciation that others have the same
   privileges that one desires for one's self.
3. Factors of time, place, manner, and amount of information.
4. Attempts to exclude oneself from others that may be
   voluntary and temporary and that may involve physical
   and(or) psychological exclusion.

Privacy often serves to maintain the patient's human dignity and integrity. A violation of privacy is often a violation

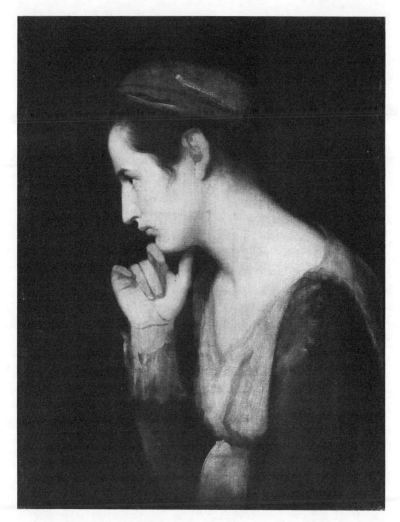

Contemplation, by George Romney. (Collection, The Denver Art Museum)

of a patient's dignity. Humiliation, embarrassment, and depersonalization often result from an invasion of privacy.

Different functions of privacy have been identified [3] :

1. Privacy maintains *personal autonomy,* one's uniqueness as a human being.

2. Privacy gives *emotional release* from the stresses and strains of day-to-day living.
3. Privacy helps in *self-evaluation,* by which one is able to examine, evaluate, and integrate one's feelings and experience. That function of privacy may be closely related to the spirituality or creative-meditative activities that bring meaning to one's life.
4. Privacy permits *limited and protected communication.* That function of privacy allows for sharing confidential information and setting boundaries and social distances in interpersonal relationships.

Obviously a number of variables affect privacy and how it manifests itself in social behavior. For example, in some African tribes there is no word or even equivalent term for privacy. Westerners have attempted to explain the concept of privacy to people in those tribes, but the concept closest to it that the people can understand is that of the hermit; that is, a private person who does not like other people or civilization. In those African cultures there are some territorial boundaries, but the concept of privacy as Westerners know it does not exist [14]. That is true also of societies in the South Pacific and in the People's Republic of China, in which privacy conflicts with the people's unity, sharing, and social welfare [13].

In spite of a wide variation of privacy norms among various cultural and social groups, there are some norms that insure a degree of individual and group privacy [29].

The support, protection, and correction often necessary for privacy is an important carative factor for the nurse. She or he must consider the functions that privacy performs for people in general and for the individual. The basic rights of the individual include privacy. The nurse recognizes those basic rights for others as well as herself or himself.

Explicit opportunities for privacy must be acknowledged in routine health experiences and in the daily care of persons, regardless of setting. Privacy consideration must include physiological and physical exposure as well as the confidentiality of limited and protected communication.

Professional integrity and confidentiality are integral parts of privacy concerns. A helping-trust relationship is often dependent on that aspect of maintaining human dignity.

Supporting a person's right to privacy can often instill in the patient faith and hope-trust in the nurse provided that privacy does not interfere with the helping therapeutic process necessary for health care. A nurse can respect the need for confidentiality while obtaining the necessary information for care. That is a point at which the helping relationship factor becomes critical for the practice of caring. However, the nurse must maintain sensitivity to the person's right to privacy.

Providing for a protective, private environment is often a first step toward other therapeutic interactions that promote or maintain health or help with care when someone is ill. Privacy interventions include information, emotional release, providing a setting for self-evaluation, and responding to the basic dignity of a person as a human being.

Both the physical and the psychological features of privacy become important considerations in the provision of a supportive, protective, or corrective environment. Likewise, privacy includes mental, physical, sociocultural, and spiritual parts that affect the meaning of privacy for each person and contribute to appropriate privacy measures.

SAFETY

Safety is a basic feature of the nurse's role. Safety concerns affect activities that the nurse performs that support, protect, or correct the environment.

Maslow identified safety as a need basic to human growth and development [15]. Safety is considered an emergent need from infancy on, and it follows a child's negotiation of confidence that his or her physiological needs will be gratified. To feel safe means to experience the absence of threat or danger. The danger threat may be perceived to be in either the internal or external environment.

When a person is young, ill, or otherwise dependent, other people (often nurses) are responsible for providing a supportive, protective, or corrective environment. Often a person's health-illness behavior may be motivated by attempts to feel safe in an environment that is unknown, depersonalized, or perceived as threatening. In addition to the external environment, the unknowns of the person's health-illness concerns or worries threaten internal safety.

Throughout a person's lifetime, he or she develops patterns of thought and action that help to explore the environment and determine whether it is safe or unsafe. Depending on previous experiences and the fulfillment of the person's safety needs, he or she will behave in a variety of ways that lead to a sense of safety. The ways of feeling safe range from a child's carrying a baby blanket everywhere to an adult's carefully checking all the doors before going to bed.

The nurse's concern for safety includes knowledge, appreciation, and tolerance of the behavior that makes a person feel psychologically safe. However, much of the nurse's practice activities are concerned with the physical components of safety. Accidents are a leading cause of death among persons in all age groups. Maintaining safety is especially crucial in caring for persons who are ill, excited, anxious, or experiencing a loss of control over their environments. Common changes that accompany illness, such as weakness, sensory deprivation, sensory overload, or incapacitation, require a person to modify his or her usual activities and ways of responding to the environment.

The nurse must be especially alert to safety factors in the environment as well as to variables that predict or cause safety threats [20] (for example, age, state of mobility, arrangement of furniture, sensory deficits, orientation, disorientation, restraining devices, and prosthetic and other supportive devices). Basic safety measures include the control of infection (e.g., by handwashing, skin care, isolation techniques, cleaning methods, and sterilization practices).

Common dangers during infancy and childhood are injuries or health problems caused by falls, burns, inhalation of foreign objects, dangerous toys, poisoning, suffocation, drowning, lack of health supervision, and lack of immunizations. The nurse should know safety measures for the adolescent that are related to driver education, community safety programs, water safety instruction, emergency care, drug use, and birth control.

During the young adult and maturity stages of life, safety concerns include industrial work conditions, (e.g., automation, toxic fumes, emotional work stress, high noises, unpleasant surroundings, isolation, and monotony). Deaths by drowning and motor vehicle accidents continue to rank high in lists of adult deaths, along with the fractures, dislocations, lacerations abrasions and contusions that often result from motor or on-the-job accidents [21].

For the older person, safety becomes a vital concern, often because of decreased mobility and impaired sensory input. In addition, common hazards in the home especially endanger an older person (as well as others of all ages); for example, slippery rugs, slick bath tubs, careless use of cigarettes and gas burners, and spilled food or other hazards on the floor. A plan for taking medications is especially important if the person has memory lapses or is disoriented.

In incorporating carative factor No. 8 into the practice of the science of caring, it is important for the nurse to (1) eliminate existing and potential hazards by arranging a safe environment, (2) explain safety precautions and procedures to the person and the family, and (3) supervise their safety precautions. The person's environmental stimuli should be adjusted and varied as necessary to prevent sensory isolation or sensory overload.

The person's environment should be arranged so that the person has as much control over it as possible and can do things for herself or himself. Availability and accessibility to others for assistance should be arranged.

Safety considerations in the environment are critical health features that are largely confined to the nurse's domain of assessment and health promotion. Carative factor No. 8 through supportive, protective, or corrective safety activities helps the nurse to develop and practice the science of caring for people of all ages.

CLEAN-ESTHETIC SURROUNDINGS

Clean-esthetic surroundings are a basic element of carative factor No. 8. The testimony of nursing history attributes major caring behaviors to that element alone. Even at a time

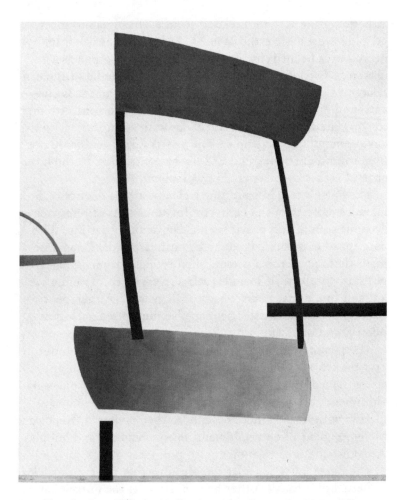

Equilibre, by Jean Hélion. (Collection, The Denver Art Museum)

when nursing care was primarily custodial, the importance of clean surroundings was never overlooked. For that reason the concept clean is linked with the concept esthetic for a better understanding of the components of care. A clean, sterile environment can often be harmful to health promotion. A personalized, pleasant, esthetic environment is appreciated by almost everyone.

There is often a need for order and symmetry and for clo-sure and completion of an act. That need helps determine esthetic nusing activities related to care. In some instances, people have a basic esthetic need [16]. Their health is improved by a beautifying of their surroundings, much as a person feels good about himself or herself when he or she can relate to the social environment. If the environment is pleasant, it will improve the affective state of the person. Attempts to correlate associations and feelings with color show how the environment affects people. The use of various colors in hospital rooms, corridors, and bed linens contributes to the influence of esthetics on a person's well-being.

The nurse's role in providing a clean-esthetic environment includes more than the basic comfort measures of removing noxious stimuli and providing a clean, sanitary setting. The concept of esthetics includes a beautification of the environment that appeals to a person's higher sense of mental and physical comfort. It includes attractiveness, color, and a pleasant and functional arrangement of furniture. A therapeutic milieu that includes esthetics can also incorporate art, music, poetry, and literature.

The pleasantness of one's surrounding helps one to interpret the world. One's self-concept and self-worth can be strengthened by an improvement in the esthetics of one's environment that contribute to comfort as well as to a satisfaction with life. Esthetics facilitate the making of friends and the enjoyment of entertainment, music, reading, and hobbies. A clean-esthetic environment also promotes a good mood.

The nurse must consider the meaning that the concept clean-esthetic holds for the other person, because the nurse's values may differ from the other person's. Nevertheless, a clean-esthetic environment usually promotes the general well-being of a person if the means to obtain it are not so compulsive that sterility results and not so obsessive that the person's privacy, comfort, and life-style are interrupted.

The purpose of the provision of a supportive, protective, or corrective environment is quality health care. Cleanliness and esthetics are closely linked with quality, in that attention to them promotes a high level of self-worth and dignity. To appeal to the higher levels in oneself and others is a worthy goal for health indeed; to actualize that component of care may promote self-actualization or gratification of the higher order needs of human beings. Esthetics can contribute to one's tastes and value system for individualization, growth, and higher development. However, esthetics cannot be gratifying if lower order needs (e.g., for cleanliness, safety, comfort, and privacy) are not gratified.

Such a basic aspect of care as cleanliness and esthetics promotes gratification of both lower and higher order needs. The carative factor discussed in the following chapters discusses the concept of lower order and higher order needs.

The discussion in this chapter identified the major external variables that help the nurse in provision of a supportive, protective, or corrective environment for the other person. The relevant concepts developed were stress-change, comfort, safety, privacy, and clean-esthetic surroundings. A holistic view was acknowledged, with emphasis on the physical, mental, sociocultural, and spiritual aspects of a person's environment.

REFERENCES

1. Arnold, M. B. *Emotion and Personality,* vol. 2. New York: Columbia University Press, 1960.
2. Beland, I. *Clinical Nursing* (2nd ed.). New York: Macmillan, 1970.
3. Bloch, D. Privacy. In C. Carlson (coordinator), *Behavioral Concepts and Nursing Intervention.* Philadelphia: Lippincott, 1970.
4. Graham, D. T., and Stevenson, I. Disease As Response to Life Stress. In H. I. Lief, V. F. Lief, and N. R. Lief (eds.), *The Psychological Basis of Medical Practice.* New York: Harper & Row, 1963.
5. Guralnik, D. (ed.). *Webster's New World Dictionary of the American Language* (2nd college ed.). New York: World, 1972.
6. Hinkle, L. The Effect of Exposure to Cultural Change, Social Change, and Changes in Interpersonal Relationships on Health. In B. S. Dohrenwend and B. P. Dohrenwend, (eds.), *Stressful Life Events.* New York: Wiley, 1974, P. 42.
7. Hinkle, L. E., Jr., Christenson, W. N., Kane, F. D., et al. An investigation of the relation between life experience, personality characteristics and general susceptibility to illness. *Psychosomatic Medicine* 20:278, 1958
8. Holmes, T. H., and Masuda, M. Life Change and Illness Susceptibility. In B. S. Dohrenwend and B. P. Dohrenwend (eds.), *Stressful Life Events.* New York: Wiley, 1974.

9. Holmes, T. H., and Rahe, R. H. The social readjustment rating scale. *Journal of Psychosomatic Research* 11:213, 1967.
10. Hudgens, R. W. Personal Catastrophe and Depression. In B. S. Dohrenwend and B. P. Dohrenwend (eds.), *Stressful Life Events.* New York: Wiley, 1974.
11. Jacox, A. Pain Research. Paper read at the Sigma Theta Tau Research Symposium, held in May, 1976, at the Molly McGee Motel in Denver, Colorado.
12. Lazarus, R. S., and Alfert, E. Short-circuiting of threat by experimentally altering cognitive appraisal. *Journal of Abnormal and Social Psychology* 69:195, 1964.
13. Lee, D. *Freedom and Culture.* Englewood Cliffs, N. J.: Prentice-Hall, 1959.
14. Personal communication (Peace Corps volunteer). The Mende of Sierra Leone. Summer, 1977.
15. Maslow, A. H. A theory of human motivation. *Psychological Review* 50:370, 1943.
16. Maslow, A. H. *Motivation and Personality.* New York: Harper & Bros., 1954.
17. Maslow, A. H. *Toward a Psychology of Being.* Princeton, N. J.: Van Nostrand, 1968.
18. Masuda, M., and Holmes, T. H. Magnitude estimations of social readjustments. *Journal of Psychosomatic Research* 11:219, 1967.
19. Mechanic, D. Discussion of Research Programs on Relations Between Stressful Life Events and Episodes of Physical Illness. In B. S. Dohrenwend and B. P. Dohrenwend (eds.), *Stressful Life Events.* New York: Wiley, 1974.
20. Mitchell, P. H. *Concepts Basic to Nursing.* New York: McGraw-Hill, 1973.
21. Murray, R., and Zentner, J. *Nursing Assessment and Health Promotion Through the Life Span.* Englewood Cliffs, N. J.: Prentice-Hall, 1975.
22. Murray, R., and Zentner, J. *Nursing Concepts for Health Promotion.* Englewood Cliffs, N.J.: Prentice-Hall, 1975.
23. Paykel, E. S. Life Stress and Psychiatric Disorder. In B. S. Dohrenwend and B. P. Dohrenwend (eds.), *Stressful Life Events.* New York: Wiley, 1974.
24. Querido, A. Forecast and follow-up. An investigation into the clinical, social, and mental factors determining the results of hospital treatment. *British Journal of Preventive and Social Medicine* 13:33, 1959.
25. Rahe, R. H., Mahan, J. L., and Arthur, R. J. Prediction of near-future health change from subjects' preceding life changes. *Journal of Psychosomatic Research* 14:401, 1970.
26. Stevens, S. S. A metric for the social consensus. *Science* 151:530, 1966.

27. Stevenson, I., and Graham, D. T. Disease As Response to Life Stress: Obtaining the Evidence Clinically. In H. I. Lief, V. F. Lief, and N. R. Lief (eds.), *The Psychological Basis of Medical Practice.* New York: Harper & Row, 1963.
28. Theorell, T. Life Events Before and After the Onset of a Premature Myocardial Infarction. In B. S. Dohrenwend and B. P. Dohrenwend (eds.), *Stressful Life Events.* New York: Wiley, 1974.
29. Westin, A. F. *Privacy and Freedom.* New York: Atheneum, 1967.
30. Wyler, A. R., Masuda, M., and Holmes, T. H. Magnitude of Life events and seriousness of illness. *Psychosomatic Medicine* 33:115, 1971.

II. ASSISTANCE WITH THE GRATIFICATION OF HUMAN NEEDS

Assistance with the gratification of human needs involves a great deal of information and subparts. For that reason the discussion of it occupies Part II of this book entirely, even though conceptually it is only one broad carative factor.

The basic human needs can be purposefully discussed from a psychosomatic or psychophysiological perspective. It is believed that such a perspective can be most useful in understanding the primary and secondary aspects of each need. A psychophysiological view is also consistent with contemporary studies of the effect of stress on the body. The dynamic, symbolic meanings and concerns of human needs are easily understood from an interactional perspective, and direct nursing care. A more common approach to human needs can be found in traditional medical surgical nursing textbooks, and it may provide a useful reference to the work here. The student nurse and the practicing nurse should refer to other resources for a thorough study of the physiological aspects of each need. The discussion of needs in this book emphasizes how the emotions and other psychological forces affect the physiological needs.

Because of the nature of people and their needs it is helpful for study and research purposes to categorize the different human needs with which the nurse commonly intervenes. Human needs can be classified as lower order and higher order needs. The lower order needs are (1) the biophysical food and fluid need, (2) the elimination need, and (3) the ventilation need. Although they are lower order biophysical needs, they are developed from a holistic, more psychological perspective relevant to health care. The human activity and sexuality needs are also classified as lower order needs, but they are labeled psychophysical rather than biophysical. Although those labels are arbitrary, they can help the student nurse and the practicing nurse understand the hierarchial perspective that is inherent in human development. The lower order biophysical needs are more fundamental for survival even though they are viewed much more broadly in the discussion here. The lower order psychophysical needs suggest not only simple survival but also the satisfaction and quality of living brought about by the gratification of those needs. The label psychophysical also connotes the larger psychological mental control that is necessary for the gratification of the activity and sexuality needs. The higher order needs are designated as psychosocial. They include (1) the achievement need, (2) the affiliation need, and (3) the need for self-actualization. They emphasize the developmental human potential, maturity, and satisfaction with self and others. The higher order needs are perhaps the long-range goals and the highest sense of contribution toward which the nurse can strive.

Practice of the carative factor assistance with the gratification of human needs, combined with the other carative factors, helps gratify higher order needs and provide the essence of what nursing ultimately seeks for quality health care.

Assistance with the gratification of human needs is important to nursing's role of helping persons in their daily activities as well as facilitating their growth and development. Even though it may sound all encompassing, the major function of the practice of caring is dependent on the success or failure of helping others in their efforts to gratify their human needs.

Often attempts to gratify human needs motivate behavior. The ways of gratifying human needs are highly variable. Determining what needs are existent and important at any time is a complex issue to which nursing must continually address itself for health care.

Studying the gratification of human needs produces so many theories and so much research that it alone could be a science.

Perhaps the best approach for nursing to take in examining human needs within the context of the science of caring is a holistic-dynamic approach that synthesizes all four components

(biophysical, psychophysical, psychosocial, and intrapersonal)
in understanding individual and group motivation and adapta-
tion in health-illness.

   Any theory of motivation or adaptation relative to the
gratification of human needs that is worthy of nursing's atten-
tion must consider the greatest adaptive capacities of the
healthy person, not just the capacities of the sick person.
Nursing theories have an obligation to health; they must be-
come and remain positive in their orientation. For that reason
nursing can take the functionalism of William James and John
Dewey and the holism of Wertheimer, Goldstein, and Gestalt
psychology and fuse them with the dynamism of Freud and
Adler. The synthesis of different orientations results in a
holistic-dynamic theory that helps one understand many
health-illness behaviors that are related to the gratification of
human needs.

   A need is generally defined as a requirement of a person,
which, if supplied, relieves or diminishes immediate distress
or improves his or her immediate sense of adequacy and well-
being [5]. The assumption is that gratification of certain
human needs is necessary for growth and development [1].
Nurses usually operate on that assumption even though their
immediate goals may be more specific (to gratify a need or
needs). Sometimes the overall goal of "human need gratifica-
tion for promotion of human growth and development" gets
lost in the process of specificity of attention to certain lower
order human needs. Attending to lower order needs becomes
an end in itself and not a way to reach the larger goal. The
for what aspect of human need concerns cannot be ignored in
nursing lest nursing lose its own major goal, which is the best
health possible, or optimal health.

   The concept of optimal health is consistent with a human
need hierarchy. One of the basic assumptions for caring is
that the nurse accept a person not only as he or she is now
but also as what he or she may become. That assumption
incorporates a view and an appreciation of a person's actualities
as well as his or her potentialities. That approach allows the
ordering of human needs while retaining a holistic-dynamic
focus. Every person has needs that must be gratified in order

to grow and develop his or her potentialities. The nurse must
be able to identify and anticipate those needs that may be
important to certain health-illness-processes. However, it is
crucial for the nurse always to assess from the patient's standpoint what needs are paramount for him or her at any given
time. The nurse's objective assessment alone may not include
the assessment of the experiencing person. At the same time
certain generalizations can be made about human needs that
help in ordering and categorizing human needs for study and
practice purposes. But regardless of how human needs are
ordered or categorized, they operate interdependently. One
need can never be completely separated from another; they
operate dynamically as a whole. A discussion here of the ordering of human needs will help the nurse maintain a balance, not
excluding one need for another, but integrating them all for
holistic care. The ordering of needs that are believed to be
most relevant to nursing as the science of caring is as follows:

1. Lower Order Needs (Biophysical Needs) ⎫
   The need for food and fluid   ⎬ Survival
   The need for elimination   ⎭   Needs
   The need for ventilation

2. Lower Order Needs (Psychophysical Needs) ⎫
   The need for activity-inactivity   ⎬ Functional
   The need for sexuality   ⎭   Needs

3. Higher Order Needs (Psychosocial Needs) ⎫
   The need for achievement   ⎬ Integrative
   The need for affiliation   ⎭   Needs

4. Higher Order Need (Intrapersonal-Inter- ⎫
   personal Need)   ⎬ Growth-seeking
   The need for self-actualization   ⎭   Need

*(The needs just listed will be discussed in subsequent chapters
as content or logic dictates. It should be noted that cultural
factors affect all the needs at all levels.)*

The lower order needs are the ones that are most obvious,
traditional, and tangible. But if nursing is really concerned

*with quality care and optimal health, it must give equal atten-
tion to all the needs. When one need is affected, all the others
are affected, directly or indirectly.*

*Maslow has listed needs that he considers basic in his theory
of human motivation [1]. Although the human needs I have
listed include some from Maslow's list, there are others that
are specific to nursing. Because the needs that Maslow lists
are so common — and relevant to nursing — I have included an
illustration that compares Maslow's hierarchy of needs to the
human needs that are important for nursing as the science of
caring.*

*Both illustrations depict the needs in a hierarchy with self-
actualization at the highest point. In the nursing hierarchy,
Maslow's physiological needs are specified, and various needs
that Maslow lists are included or subsumed under other,
broader needs; for example, love-belongingness is a part of
the affiliation need. I think that the need for self-actualization is the highest level need.*

*The practice of nursing as the science of caring demands
that the nurse respond to the patient as an individual. In so
doing, the nurse assists with the gratification of the patient's
needs. Once a patient is recognized, appreciated, and treated
as an individual, he or she has more energy to move up the
hierarchy of needs toward self-actualization.*

*Regardless of their hierarchical status, human needs are
complex, and they have different meanings and purposes for
different individuals and groups. Meeting only lower order
needs may not help a person toward optimal health. Attention must be given to higher order needs as well.*

*In the development and practice of assistance with the
gratification of human needs, a useful approach is to view the
needs as belonging to and affecting individuals, not as isolated
concerns. In other words, the whole person may be in need,
not just parts of the body (e.g., the stomach, intestines, geni-
tals, or musculoskeletal system). Certain needs may only be
part of a larger need, and not ends in themselves (e.g., the
human need for affiliation may be a part of a need to be
accepted and loved).*

Keeping in mind the holistic-dynamic framework for

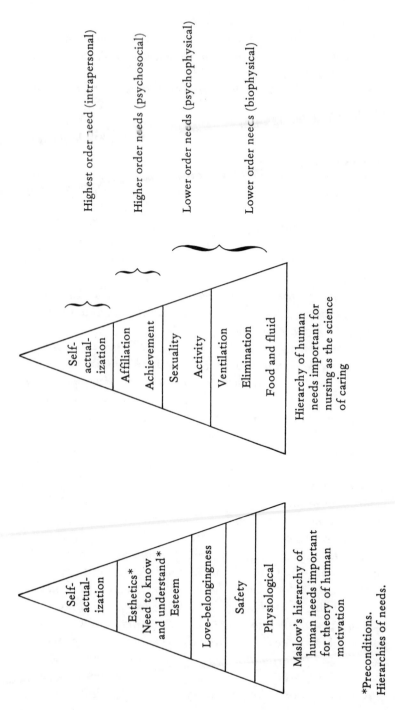

Highest order need (intrapersonal)

Higher order needs (psychosocial)

Lower order needs (psychophysical)

Lower order needs (biophysical)

Self-actualization

Affiliation
Achievement

Sexuality
Activity

Ventilation
Elimination
Food and fluid

Hierarchy of human needs important for nursing as the science of caring

Self-actualization

Esthetics*
Need to know and understand*
Esteem

Love-belongingness

Safety

Physiological

Maslow's hierarchy of human needs important for theory of human motivation

*Preconditions.
Hierarchies of needs.

viewing human needs, the carative factor assistance with the gratification of human needs leads to a more complete development of each human need. Some needs are more familiar and concrete because of the tangible ways in which they manifest themselves. Others are more abstract and elusive. They all are equally important for quality nursing care and the promotion of optimal health. In spite of the hierarchial way in which the needs are presented, they all must be valued. Continual theoretical and clinical efforts should be made scientifically and humanistically to help people gratify their human needs. A large part of nursing's function and goals is covered by the carative factor assistance with the gratification of human needs if it is valued in its entirety and attention is paid to the abstract needs as well as the concrete needs.

REFERENCES

1. Maslow, A. H. A theory of human motivation. *Psychological Review* 50:370, 1943.
2. Maslow, A. H. *Motivation and Personality.* New York: Harper & Bros., 1954.
3. Maslow, A. H. *Toward a Psychology of Being* (2nd ed.). Princeton, N. J.: Van Nostrand, 1968.
4. Mitchell, P. H. *Concepts Basic to Nursing.* New York: McGraw-Hill, 1973.
5. Orlando, I. *The Dynamic Nurse-Patient Relationship.* New York: Putnam's, 1961.

6. ASSISTANCE WITH THE GRATIFICATION OF LOWER ORDER BIOPHYSICAL NEEDS

THE FOOD AND FLUID NEED

Food becomes symbolically equated with life, health and growth, but most especially with mother's love [5].

Although the food and fluid need is categorized as a lower order biophysical need essential for survival, its satisfaction establishes a vital foundation for a person's higher order needs related to personality and social development. The human need for food and fluid means much more than the need to survive. In all cultures, eating and food are integral parts of human social and emotional relationships from birth on. Eating is believed to be motivated more by feelings than by logic. "In most societies, food is the focus of emotional relationships, a channel for interpersonal relations, for the communication of love or discrimination or disapproval; it usually has a symbolic reference" [20].

The early mother-child feeding experience is a continuation of the prenatal symbiotic relationship with dependence-reciprocal satisfaction. The feeding relationship is the original mode of establishing a relationship with another person, and it provides the most critical opportunity for trust development.

There is in infants an in-built propensity to be in touch with and to cling to a human being. In this sense there is a "need" for an object independent of food which is as primary as the need for food . . . [5].

The individual from birth on does not simply ingest food and fluid. Significant other things (the experience and associated sensations, the surroundings) become incorporated into the body and into the developing personality through feeding and eating.

Oral activities, eating behavior, habits, associations, taste in food, and desires are directly associated with the meanings and relationships that have been attached to the eating process from birth on. During infancy the "good mother" through the feeding process becomes introjected into the child for purposes of identification and learning purposes. Consequently, the "good mother" associations become "good me" meanings. Therefore, the foundation and origin of self in relation to another is established during the early experiences of the gratification of the food and fluid need.

The food and fluid need is foremost during the first developmental stage of life. The basic food and fluid need originates as a lower order need to survive as the child enters the world in a state of helplessness. The child's world revolves around hunger and its satisfaction. The child's discomforts are either removed or not removed. Gratification of the food and fluid need depends entirely on the external human environment.

The higher order meanings and associations connected with food and fluid need depend on the quality of early and continuing symbolic associations of the eating experience. In essence the gratification of food and fluid need depends on love, security, and trust as much as on nutritional requirements. The amount of food or the fact that it is provided does not determine gratification. It is misleading to label the need for food and fluid as a human need without explaining that the *secondary aspects* of the intake of nutrients are *primary* requirements for survival and future development. Food and fluid and their symbolic and related human relationship components are crucial to psychological and sociocultural health as well as to physical existence.

Eating habits and tastes in food vary from culture to culture. In the United States, the cultural basis of eating habits is important in understanding another person's food and fluid needs. The United States is a multicultural nation. Eating habits depend on cultural or religious experiences. Food can be part of a familiar environment that is soothing and promotes security and contentment. The nurse must be knowledgeable and appreciative of the need to include culturally valued foods into nutritional programs. Depending on one's cultural or religious experiences, different foods or tastes in food are valued or prohibited. Different cultures place significance on different foods. For example, in the Southwestern United States, beans, tortillas, and highly seasoned foods are commonly eaten. In the South, fat pork, hot breads, and grits are commonly eaten. In the Midwest, steak and beef are commonly eaten. Just as people in different parts of the United States or different cultural groups in the United States have their own eating habits, so do different nations. Pork is forbidden in Moslem countries. Hindus do not eat beef. In the United States many people have turned to a vegetarian diet, which is considered nutritionally sound.

Recent social and cultural trends in the United States show a change in the meaning and selection of foods. Many young and older adults are interested in "health foods," natural grains, vegetables, and a nonmeat diet.

Often the selection of food and certain diets (e.g., a vegetarian diet or a high-meat diet) is associated with a certain status or group. People who make a lot of money usually eat steak and other meats; youths and young adults are interested in low-meat or nonmeat diets. To one person, a food may be unfit to eat, to another a delicacy. One's attitude often depends on one's sociocultural experiences and conditioning.

The values of a country or a subgroup in the country often motivate people to eat or not eat. Most people do not eat to be healthy; they eat for satisfaction, contentment, and good feelings. Eating and drinking are universal signs of friendship and goodwill.

Food is also symbolically associated with health and beauty; for example, some people think that plumpness is beautiful and healthy, whereas others believe that slimness is beautiful and healthy.

The psychological feelings associated with the intake of food and fluid are not divorced from the physical effects of eating. Physically, there is an internal warmth as food is swallowed. The bodily processes and sensations of eating occur in the lips, mouth, and tongue. Those areas are the most sensitive, pleasurable, and soothing regions of the body. Through the act of feeding, the infant experiences many

primary and secondary sources of pleasure. The stimulation
of the mouth, the acts of sucking and swallowing, and the
cuddling against a warm body are all aspects of the satisfaction and development of the food and fluid need.

Within the context of the science of caring, a holistic-
dynamic approach should be used in assessing, planning, intervening in, and evaluating food and fluid need for nursing care.
A scientific research base exists that helps confirm the dynamic
state of the emotions that are associated with food and fluid.
A holistic approach must be used to link accurately the behavioral and biophysical processes that are related to gratification
of the food and fluid need. The literature reveals a dynamic
interplay between the biophysical, emotional, and behavioral
aspects of the need for food and fluid that are associated with
health-illness disturbances. The major aspects and the disturbances related to them are listed to help students and practitioners gain knowledge and awareness of the holistic significance
of the food and fluid need.

Health-Illness Disturbances That Are Associated
with the Food and Fluid Need
Biophysical Aspects of the Food and Fluid Need. A system
of the body that serves a biological need can be diverted from
its original purpose to serve a physical-psychological need.
The diversion can cause a physical or a psychological compensation by the biological system used. The compensation diminishes the amount of energy available for balance. The system
cannot adequately serve both needs, and somatic-physical
bodily changes or illness can result. For example, the eating
process and the system that is necessary for biophysical maintenance and survival can be used to deal with a psychological
need, such as the need for security. The disorders that result
have emotional roots that affect the organs and viscera, and
they are primarily biophysical.

Various approaches can help one to understand the holistic
relationship between the primary and secondary aspects of
food and fluid. They range from those of Freud, Cannon,
Alexander, French, and Wolf to the more modern, dynamic
approaches related to stress-change.

Some theorists think that emotions are derived from biological processes. For example, Plutchik [23] thought that
emotions were adaptive devices that have played a role in
survival at all stages of evolution. A prototype of an adaptive
behavior pattern and the emotions associated with it are
shown in Table 6-1.

Table 6-1. Emotions Associated with Adaptive Behavior Patterns

Prototype of an Adaptive Behavior Pattern	Primary Emotion
Incorporation: Ingestion of food and water	Acceptance
Rejection-riddance: Excretion, vomiting	Disgust
Destruction: Removal of barrier to satisfaction	Anger
Protection: Response to pain or threats of pain or harm	Fear
Reproduction: Sexual responses	Joy
Deprivation: Loss of pleasurable object that has been contacted or incorporated into one's self	Sorrow
Orientation: Response to contact with new or strange object	Startle
Exploration: Random exploration of environment	Expectation or curiosity

There has been much confusion and controversy in the
literature over the concept of "psychosomatic" or psychophysiological conditions. Recently there has been some appreciation of holistic care and a trend toward that approach.

There exists a complex interrelationship between psychological states and physiological functions. However, some confusion still exists. Even in nursing, which has always been
holistic, there is the tendency to respond to the obvious
dimensions that each human need encompasses rather than to
study more the dynamic, symbolic aspects of each need for a
more complete, holistic approach to the practice of caring.

The current thinking about holistic care emphasizes (1) that
etiological components that have many factors interact and
produce change through complex neurophysiological and

neurochemical pathways, (2) that each psychological function has a physiological correlate, and (3) that each physiological function has a psychological correlate.

Some of the most common disturbances in health-illness that are associated with the need for food and fluid are briefly discussed here as examples of complex etiologies with many factors. One who is concerned with holistic care cannot separate the etiological dimensions.

Common Disturbances in Health-Illness. Anorexia, dysphagia, pica, and bulimia are believed to be closely related to frustration or nongratification of the need for food and fluid. Common examples of health-illness conditions that occur during adulthood and are closely associated with (or at least affected by) the food and fluid need are diabetes, peptic ulcer, gastritis, anorexia nervosa, and alcoholism. Those conditions are often associated with behavioral problems related to eating, such as dependency, anxiety, and diet control.

The following are brief descriptions of the conditions associated with the food and fluid need:

Bulimia is characterized by an inordinate appetite and excessive eating that may lead to obesity and secondary medical problems.

Dysphagia is the inability to swallow. It may be neurophysical in origin.

Anorexia nervosa is characterized by a loss of appetite so severe that it may threaten life. The condition is thought to symbolize the expulsion or rejection of a love object and to result from frustrations associated with a disturbed relationship with a love object during the feeding experiences of infancy.

Gastritis ("nervous stomach") is characterized by gastric distress and pain. It may start with vomiting.

A *peptic ulcer* is a lesion of the mucous lining of the stomach or duodenum (duodenal ulcer).

Pica refers to the eating of a nonnutritive substance, such as chalk or paper.

An early, classic experiment illustrated the holistic relationship between the biophysical response and the emotions

associated with the intake of food [8]. Three men were hyp-
notized, and each was told that when he awakened he would
find a bar of chocolate on the table beside him, and that he
would have an irresistible desire to eat it. Each man was also
told that since the chocolate did not belong to him, it would
be wrong to eat it. The responses of each person when he
awakened were reported as follows:

1. Person 1 had a negative hallucination. He did not see the
   candy, and so he avoided the conflict by denial or repression.
2. Person 2 manifested signs of acute anxiety accompanied
   by neurocirculatory collapse. He became dizzy, faint, and
   unable to walk; he was pale and cold and had a rapid pulse.
3. Person 3 showed outward composure and talked about
   food and eating, remarking that visitors were expected to
   accept food. He ate the chocolate. But in a few minutes,
   the chocolate tasted bitter to him. He complained of pain
   and nausea, and then he vomited.

The study demonstrates that many factors affect the ingestive process and the holistic gratification of the food and fluid
need.

Alexander and French [3] reported that emotions such as
fear, anger, resentment, guilt, and embarrassment have definite
physical effects. They reported that even though everyone
experiences transitory emotional states that affect bodily processes, sustained emotional strain may lead to chronic disturbances of biophysical functions.

In analyzing those findings, the nurse must keep a holistic-
dynamic focus in helping the other person with gratification
of the food and fluid need. Keeping such a focus is not as
simple as it may seem.

Research findings have established that emotional conflict
is one of the critical factors associated with physical disorders.
A holistic focus must be acknowledged with any preventive
modality or treatment in the science of caring. At the same
time it is important to note that almost all the research relating
emotional factors to biophysical conditions used correlational

studies. The word *cause* was used in the reports, but it must be remembered that correlation does not mean causation. Correlation means the factors are closely associated; but the cause is not necessarily one or another of the associated factors. Common conditions that have many possible causes are ulcer, anorexia nervosa, diabetes and obesity. They all involve gratification of the food and fluid need.

The illness associated with the food and fluid need that has been most intensively studied is *peptic ulcer*. Peptic ulcers have always been more common in men than in woman (but that incidence may be changing). Peptic ulcers often develop in a person who has a history of chronic gastric distress, a condition that results from chronic gastric spasm, gastric overactivity, and overeating. In gastritis there is an oversecretion of the hydrochloric acid in the stomach, even when there is no food present to absorb the excess acid. The acid irritates and inflames the mucous lining of the stomach or duodenum, and an ulcer forms.

Peptic ulcer has been described psychodynamically as a disease in which the "hungry stomach eats itself [1]." The ulcer symbolizes a longing for love shown by the craving for food. It is interesting to note that ulcer pain is relieved by food and aggravated by hunger.

Sullivan [30] described the "ulcer personality" after a review of literature and a clinical study of 200 peptic ulcer patients. Typically, the person with an ulcer is tense, driving, restless, pleasant and likeable, successful, responsible, sexually well-adjusted, striving for superiority, competitive, overextended in activities, and insecure.

Alexander [1, 2] in his psychoanalyses of persons with ulcers found that the desire for rest, comfort, support, and loving care existed in ulcer patients who appeared on the surface to be ambitious, hard-driving, and competitive.

Dependency and aggression are commonly occurring behaviors in persons with peptic ulcer. Alexander felt that perhaps the dependency longing that is linked with loving care and the receiving of food (in infancy) becomes suppressed in the person with an ulcer and a chronic state of tension results. The tension in turn activates the digestive process.

The aggression has been explained psychodynamically as being associated with frustration of the desire for food and angry crying during infancy. According to that explanation, the emotions do not go away with time, and the hostility and anger from infancy affect the adult's digestive system. Tension, anger, and resentment have been widely reported to be accompanied by increase in the secretion of hydrochloric acid, mucus, and pepsin.

Symptoms of an ulcer have been reported to disappear when anger and hostility have been expressed openly and to reappear under conditions of competitive career striving [33]. There are many different explanations for ulcers, but for the purposes of this book, it is important that the reader be made aware of the complexity of the causes of one condition, such as the ulcer. Because of that complexity, it is incumbent on nurses to take a holistic-dynamic approach in assistance with the gratification of the food and fluid need. Such a holistic approach is expecially relevant in caring for a person who has an ulcer.

Anorexia nervosa is another illness that is often associated with the food and fluid need. The condition is more common in women than in men. A negative attitude toward food and the resulting lack of appetite has often been associated with anxiety and guilt attached to food and the eating and feeding processes. The attitude may be secondary to other conditions.

Some of the common causes of anorexia nervosa that are attached to the human food and fluid need are:

1. Rejection of a love object, self-punishment or even suicidal intentions and punishment of others or of society in general
2. Resistance to advancing to higher levels of development (such as from adolescence to adulthood)
3. Anxiety about one's sexual development
4. Unconscious fear of oral impregnation based on misconceptions and distortions of sexuality need
5. Aggressive resistance to parental demands

Those views and associations indicate that physical disorders of the ingestive process can originate during the oral period of infancy. They suggest that the food and fluid need expressed during infancy affects adult life. The frustrations associated with the early feeding process in infancy (e.g., a poor supply of milk, the desire to nurse rather than to be weaned, the sense of rejection by one's mother) become critical developmental issues that are thought to manifest themselves later in many ways (e.g., behaviorally, such as by mistrust, or biophysically, such as in an eating disorder). The child who refuses to eat or who vomits after most feedings usually has experienced severe frustration or rejection during feedings. The behavior reflects the home environment and maternal relationship. The child is attempting to get rid of the unpleasantness of the environment (the people) that has been incorporated with the meal. The feeling of expulsion and sickness associated with an unpleasant eating situation can be carried through life.

Diabetes is another illness associated with the food and fluid need. Some researchers support the theory that diabetes is caused by psychological-social factors, especially by emotional stress. It has not been demonstrated conclusively that psychological or social stress causes diabetes, but there is sufficient evidence to indicate a close association between stressful events and diabetes onset. Regardless of its cause, the disorder and its treatment directly affect the person's food and fluid need. The restricted diet often produces the following reactions:

1. Extreme compulsiveness in adhering to the diet (rigid self-restriction may ward off anxiety).
2. Complete violation of the diet, with deliberate, systematic overeating. That behavior may be self-punishment related to guilt about having the disorder. It may suggest to the nurse that the patient has a distortion of the meaning or cause of the illness. Violating the diet may be a way of punishing others. The violation may be especially evident in an adolescent who is attempting to emancipate himself or herself from parental restrictions. The increased assertiveness or rebelliousness about the diet and treatment may be a weapon used against parents or others. It can be used as a means of controlling relationships.

3. Difficulty with the postponement of pleasure — a person
   may neglect his or her diet for the immediate pleasure of
   fulfilling a need. There may also be a secondary gain of
   attention. For example, attention from parents or others,
   such as health professionals, regarding diet control may
   serve as a source of indirect satisfaction for a person, even
   though the attention may be negative. Such a habitual
   mode of behavior becomes a source of gain that is secondary to illness or disease process, but serves a psychological
   function for the person. When one's diet is restricted, one
   tends to become preoccupied with food. Also, one often
   has an intense desire to eat when one is bored, lonely, un-
   loved, or angry. Eating can provide temporary relief of
   feelings. That is one of the reasons the biophysical need
   for food and fluid gets confused with deeper emotional
   needs and requires that the nurse view the food and fluid
   need comprehensively.

   Obesity is a frequently occurring health problem that is
obviously associated with gratification of the food and fluid
need. Obesity is often defined as the condition of being more
than 20 percent overweight. It results from an excessive accumulation of fatty tissue. Twenty to 25 percent of adults and
10 percent of school-aged children are overweight [4]. Obesity
is a growing public health problem that is found all over the
world. It is a major concern because it has an adverse effect
on health and life expectancy. (Diabetes is thought to be
closely associated with obesity.) The mortality rates are higher
among persons who are overweight.
   In spite of the health problems associated with obesity,
treatment of the condition is generally unsuccessful. The literature indicates that only two percent of dieters lose sufficient
weight and maintain a desirable weight. Many people lose
weight, but they find it difficult to keep the weight off [20,
29]. Complex interactions of many factors determine obesity
and its outcome, and thus the food and fluid need of an obese
person is particularly complicated. A holistic-dynamic approach
to assistance with gratification of the food and fluid need
and with health care in general is vital. Nursing care must

include a plan that involves the participation of the person
and an understanding of the dynamics of eating behavior. The
interpersonal and emotional support related to assistance with
the gratification of the food and fluid need of an obese person
must be great. The success of various weight control groups
that offer interpersonal pressure and support attests to the
effectiveness of a holistic approach. Nutritional instruction,
diet planning, and exercise classes alone are almost totally
ineffective. The person needs help to gain control over the
dominant aspect of the food and fluid need or to develop a
different way to meet certain components of the food and
fluid need.

Assistance with gratification of the food and fluid need
plays a role in every — or almost every — nursing care situation.
The food and fluid need is inherent in the etiology of many
illnesses, and it affects a person's recovery from almost all of
them. For that reason, it may be helpful to summarize the
significance of the carative factor assistance with the gratification of the food and fluid need.

Significance of the Food and Fluid Need for
the Practice of Caring

1. Theory and research support the clinical proposition that
   emotion is one of the critical factors associated with biophysical disorders of the ingestive process that are related
   to the food and fluid need. The emotional factors can
   create an imbalance or precede the onset of an illness or
   affect its course.
2. Empirical data have established a multifactorial basis for
   disorders related to gratification of the food and fluid
   need.
3. Oversimplication, or singling out one factor as *the* cause
   of a health-illness condition, should be avoided. A holistic-
   dynamic approach is more effective for nursing care.
4. The food and fluid need suggests much more than the
   intake of nourishment for survival and the minimum daily
   requirements of foods:
   a. The food and fluid need is associated with trust, love,

warmth, and security in human relationships.
b. The food and fluid need is associated with dependency strivings.
c. The food and fluid need is directly related to past experiences, the conscious and unconscious, symbolic and real meanings attached to the feeding process.
d. The intake of food and fluid is associated with one's self-concept and image.
5. The carative factor assistance with gratification of the food and fluid need is perhaps the most basic and symbolic of all carative factors.
6. The practice of the science of caring must include an understanding of people's desires, likes, and felt needs to eat, an appreciation of what eating and food mean to a person.
7. The cultural significance of food habits must be incorporated into a plan of caring. Familiar foods give people a sense of security. The practice of caring must be attentive to the food and fluid need and use a holistic approach.
8. More and more researchers believe that eating is motivated by feelings, not by logic. Food is a focus of emotional associations and a channel for interpersonal relationships.
9. The establishment of eating habits begins at birth; one's culture and past experiences define for one what is edible and how and under what circumstances foods are to be eaten, savored, or valued.
10. To effectively assist another person with gratification of the food and fluid need, it is necessary for nursing to develop a holistic-dynamic approach to the relevant study, practice, and research activities.

THE ELIMINATION NEED
Assistance with the elimination need is an essential carative factor in nursing. The elimination need includes many external environmental events as well as internal subjective feeling states. It includes concepts of privacy, meaning of bodily functions, toilet habits, and the relationship between a person's internal feeling state and physical sensations.

The elimination need is biological, and it is related to the maintenance of a normal metabolic and homeostatic balance between the external and internal environments. Nurses often help patients establish normal excretory functions and patterns. Because of the subjective way a person looks at the act of helping to gratify the elimination need, it is necessary to consider the feelings and associations that are part of gratification of that need.

According to Freud, Erikson, and others, the psychological origin of assistance with gratification of the elimination need begins with the beginning of the toilet-training process and the developmental stage of autonomy as opposed to shame and doubt. As a child enters the bowel and bladder-training stages (around 18 months to 3½ years of age) the erogenous zone of the child's body shifts from the mouth (which permits sucking and oral fulfillment) to the anus and elimination. During the first year or two of life, the child has been completely dependent and has been the *receiver*. Now the parents' expectation is that the child become the *giver*. In terms of internal bodily perceptions, the child would rather defecate whenever he or she feels tension in the lower intestines. However, social and parental standards do not permit that after the child has reached a certain age. The child has to conform to society's standards of cleanliness; the child has to learn to *hold in* and *let go* in accordance with the external environment rather than in accordance with the child's internal environment. The child is expected by society to move from an irresponsible state to a responsible one.

The conflict in conforming is made worse by the child's natural curiosity, explorative motivations, and pride in his or her first creation — the feces. The child's internal bodily perceptions say one thing and the external environment says another — and the child must learn to conform to society's rules. The child will of course, conform in regard to bowel activity. However, whether conformity of thoughts and feelings occurs depends on some interrelated factors, such as:

1. The mother-child relationship
2. The gratification of the food and fluid need

3. The attitude of the parents toward the child and the child's body
4. The parents' attitudes toward their bodies
5. The religious and cultural attitudes toward cleanliness, modesty, privacy, and bodily functions

The attitude of the child's parents or of the culture affects the child's ability to learn to gratify the elimination need in a constructive way. Whether a child learns a matter-of-fact approach to elimination or a compulsive, rigid, highly structured approach depends on the external environment, usually on the parents' attitude and behavior, which affect the child's feelings about elimination. The foundation is built for future attitudes and behaviors in regard to the elimination need. The nurse's assistance in gratifying the elimination need extends beyond the physical excretory function to feeling states, practices of cleanliness, privacy, ritualistic behaviors, attitudes about the body, and even one's self-concept. The development of autonomy, flexibility, curiosity, and creativity is possible during the formative years via assistance with the elimination need. The instillation of shame, doubt and rigidity, the stifling of curiosity, and the inhibition of creative expression can also occur during the early years and affect the development of a child's personality. The early parent-child relationship and the gratification of the food and fluid need determine the pattern of the rest of the parent-child relationship. The foundation is established for future development, ingrained attitudes, and associations related to the elimination need.

In the United States especially, mention of the excretory functions of the body are not socially acceptable. An attitude of privacy and embarrassment is associated with the elimination need. It seems as though people are not supposed to have such a need because of the sights, smells, or uncleanliness associated with its gratification.

Southern European and Latin American attitudes toward elimination are much more open to and accepting of elimination as a normal human function. In the United States the need is camouflaged to such an extent that it becomes regarded as something that shouldn't exist or at least not be openly

acknowledged. It is strictly a private matter. The existence
of pay toilets in the United States symbolizes an attitude
toward elimination. One does not gratify the elimination
need unless one can pay to do so. The pay toilet establishes
a barrier, and it acknowledges the privacy that the people of
the United States consider necessary for the gratification of
the elimination need. Recently human rights groups have pro-
tested pay toilets in public facilities as discriminatory. Their
existence is being challenged as a violation of human rights.
Some places are removing pay toilets, while other places are
ignoring the issue. In a "progressive" western city a debate
took place recently over whether the city should provide public toilet facilities in a shopping mall. Some people thought
that public toilets would encourage "undesirables" to loiter
on the mall. The message seems to be that only undesirables
would need to use the toilet — and that "socially desirables"
would, by reason of their money and respectability, be spared
that need.

Bathrooms in U.S. homes and hotels have a high social
value. Some Americans have labeled the bathroom the shrine.
The use of such euphemisms as bathroom, ladies' room, and
men's room indicates a reluctance to acknowledge the excretory function that takes place in the toilet.

A parent — or an entire culture — may establish values and
norms related to the gratification of the elimination need. The
Protestant ethic encourages compulsive cleanliness (cleanliness
is next to godliness). People in Western countries, especially
England and the United States, seem to have feelings of shame
and disgust in regard to elimination.

The child's mental development occurs simultaneously with
the development of the elimination need. The child is learning
to incorporate the parental and cultural attitudes and expectations toward right and wrong, toward what is acceptable and
what is unacceptable. The child introjects the wishes and
desires of the parent, making them a part of his or her own
mind. Therefore, the development of awareness of the elimination need coincides with the development of the conscience
and the superego. The child will conform to his parents' wishes
even if conforming conflicts with his or her own internal

bodily perceptions and subjective feeling states. Invariably conflict is created, but the degree of negative meanings and attitudes of severe harshness as opposed to kind firmness, patience, and positive acceptance in the parents toward elimination determines the attitude of the child toward the elimination need. Whether the child develops feelings of shame, guilt, and rigidity or of acceptance and matter-of-factness toward elimination depends on the external norms, values, and behaviors that he or she encounters.

The behaviors of dependence as opposed to independence are related to both the origin of the elimination need and the origin of the food and fluid need. The child quickly learns the delight of power and control not only over elimination (defecation and urination) but also over others as the child decides to conform or not conform.

During the psychological origin of gratification of elimination need, the child usually wants and tries to please the parents. Parents sometimes forget that children want to conform and to do what is expected of them. Parents need to believe that the child will conform. Society's views toward children often affect the parents' trust in their child's development. If society views the child as evil and bad (as Watson did in the forties), society believes the child's impulses must be controlled. In such a society, the parents' attitude and behavior toward the child are likely to be more anxious, compulsive, and rigid than if the society believes that the child is inherently good and thus can be relied on to grow and develop satisfactorily. The latter view is represented in the works of Benjamin Spock (in regard to children) and Carl Rogers (in regard to adults). A philosophy of inherent goodness or of inherent badness can affect almost all the day-to-day responses in childrearing as well as in other interpersonal situations.

When one understands the psychological origin of the elimination need, one can begin to understand the later internal perceptions, associations and subjective feeling states surrounding the elimination need, its gratification and other bodily functions. One can also begin to appreciate the possibility that certain internal feeling states affect bodily functions related to ingestion and elimination. The following paragraphs discuss major studies and views of how the subjective internal states affect elimination and the whole gastrointestinal system.

That gastrointestinal functioning can be inhibited by fear or anger was early demonstrated by Cannon [6, 7, 9]. Other observations about the gastrointestinal system that were reported later relate to differentiated responses in the stomach and the rectum that occur with pleasant and unpleasant emotions. Gastric hypofunction was associated with startle situations, fatigue, and a variety of strong feelings. Other studies reported significantly greater gastric acidity under stress, such as that connected with academic examinations [15].

Some of the most fascinating information about internal perceptions and the functioning of the gastrointestinal system has emerged from early studies of people who have had gastric fistulas. Wolf and Wolff, in particular, studied one such person over a five-year period [34]. For that person, pleasant food associations resulted in increased gastric motility, marked increases in acidity, and a darker color of the mucosa. The emotions of being overwhelmed, dejected, or angry were associated with inhibition of gastric secretions and sometimes with anorexia and nausea.

Psychological variables in gastrointestinal functioning have also been studied. Wolff, Grace, and Wolf observed patients with different kinds of colonic fistulas [36]. "Conflict, anger, resentment, and hostility" were associated with colonic *hyper*-function. Fear and dejection were associated with gastrointestinal *hypo*functioning. There are also reports that persons with hyperactive bowels who were allowed to ventilate hostile feelings felt calm and relaxed and had less active, less contracted bowels [7].

Different feeling states have been associated with different disorders of the elimination function. For example, persons with ulcerative colitis have been described as "outwardly calm, superficially peaceful, and with more than usual dependency" [7, 36]. Hostility, resentment, and guilt have been identified as the internal states that affect elimination. Other gastrointestinal conditions, such as chronic constipation, have been associated with tenseness, hostility, and rigid determination to solve one's problems. In contrast, persons with functional diarrhea have been described in the literature as soft-spoken, regressive, and infantile. Wishes for dependency and helplessness are commonly reported in association with diarrhea.

It has been postulated clinically that continual psychological bombardment of the autonomic nervous system by intense feelings may result in physical disorders, such as chronic constipation, diarrhea, or even ulcerative colitis.

The clinical studies and the psychodynamic view of disorders of the gastrointestinal system have been mentioned to point out the connection of the broader, symbolic internal perceptions of the elimination need with its biophysical aspects. A holistic view of the carative factor assistance with the gratification of the elimination need is important in the routine aspects of care for everyone. However, the broader psychological aspects of the need become even more important in caring for people who have disorders of the gastrointestinal system. Some of the disorders of elimination can get confused early in life with feelings of giving, retaining, conforming, or rebelling.

Some examples of disturbances that are thought to result from the early psychological origin of the elimination need are:

1. An *anxiety reaction* in a child who is afraid to sleep for fear of soiling.
2. *Direct functional disturbances,* such as constipation, prolonged bladder or bowel accidents after the child has been toilet trained, and receiving pleasure from enemas or suppositories as a secondary gratification.
3. *Phobias and compulsions* are related to the desire to be perfect or clean or to control and possess. They later become associated with avarice, greed, and the fear of "letting go," of losing control, or of releasing destructive forces in one's self and(or) others.

The wish to be autonomous and free from the demands and expectations of others can affect other areas of life as well as the gastrointestinal system.

The three emotions most commonly associated with elimination disorders are anxiety, guilt, and anger-resentment. The desire to express anger and hostility can cause untimely and spasmodic movements of the bowels. The wish to retain possession, control, and power over one's bowels as well as one's life can affect the colon and result in chronic constipation.

Both psychodynamic and biological perspectives are necessary for holistic understanding of the elimination need and the behaviors and meanings related to it. To practice the science of caring, one must consider the external bodily functions as well as the internal perceptions and subjective "feeling states." The carative factor assistance with the gratification of the elimination need encompasses psychological associations and coping as well as complex and subtle sociocultural variables, such as privacy, modesty, and morality.

Significance of the Elimination Need for the Practice of Caring

1. Psychophysiological theory and research support the clinical proposition that subjective "feeling states" and internal perceptions are associated with bodily functions and physical disorders of the elimination system.
2. Assistance with the gratification of the elimination need suggests much more than biophysical defecation and urination:
   a. The elimination need may be associated with feelings of anxiety, anger, guilt, possession, resentment, control, and dependency.
   b. Attitudes toward the elimination need are associated with societal-cultural views toward children (e.g., are children good or evil?) and attitudes toward cleanliness, modesty, privacy, morality, immorality, and toilet habits.
   c. The elimination need is directly related to one's experiences and to one's conscious and unconscious perceptions, meanings, and feelings (real or symbolic) attached to the elimination process.
   d. Gratification of the elimination need is associated with future personality development, and it can affect one's self-concept, body image, and bodily functions.

3. The practice of caring must include an understanding of people's desires, habits, ideas of and associations with the elimination need.

4. The cultural and personal significance of elimination habits must be incorporated into a plan of caring.

5. Elimination habits and other aspects of the elimination need are established from approximately 18 months of age on; one's personal, cultural, and social beliefs define what is acceptable and how and under what circumstances the elimination need is to be met.

6. The elimination need is biological in nature, but the feelings and associations related to gratification of the need pervade many other aspects of one's life, habits, attitudes, and behaviors.

7. The elimination need begins simultaneously with the development of the child's mental apparatus, conscience, and superego functions. Therefore, parental and societal attitudes regarding elimination are incorporated into the child's mind during that stage and they affect future development.

8. The child wants and tries to please his or her parents by conforming, even though conforming can create varying degrees of conflict with the child's internal bodily perceptions and subjective feeling states.

9. During the early stages of the development of the elimination need, the child can be helped to sublimate his or her drives and instincts by playing with mud, sand, play dough, clay, cookie dough, and so on.

10. The foundation for gratification of the elimination need can promote autonomy, flexibility, curiosity, and creativity, or it can promote shame, doubt, rigidity, the stifling of curiosity, and the inhibition of creativity.

11. The assistance with gratification of the elimination need is an important part of routine care for all patients. But an understanding of holistic care is far from routine; it includes a broad understanding of the elimination need, which is confused with feelings of giving, retaining, conforming, and rebelling. In caring for healthy people, as well as for people with elimination disorders, a holistic

perspective is critical for quality care. A holistic caring perspective draws on diverse scientific and clinical findings that complement nursing practices.

THE VENTILATION NEED

The ventilation need discussed in the following paragraphs includes those components of that lower order biophysical need that are related to the respiratory and circulatory systems. Biophysically those two systems are interconnected. Frequently a malfunction of one of those systems affects the other. For that reason, the two systems are often physically and biologically altered by similar psychological stimuli and environmental stresses.

Both systems can be considered as involving lower order biophysical needs for categorical purposes. However, the major focus of the discussion is on holistic social and emotional factors related to ventilation needs, which influence the health status and health care of individuals.

A broader approach to understanding illness and health maintenance is needed in this day and age, when there is an enchantment with science and technology in all aspects of health care. A holistic orientation precludes the study and practice of what can only be seen, felt, and measured by a tangible means. Research has shown that there is a high incidence of psychosomatic illness among people of all socioeconomic groups in the U.S. U.S. society has been called a psychosomatically oriented society [12]. A formal acknowledgment of the importance of psychosocial and cultural variables in understanding health-illness is necessary for everyone in the health professions.

Current social environmental stresses further affect the bodily systems that deliver oxygen and blood throughout the body. Repeated studies have shown that a large percentage of all patients receiving general medical care are suffering primarily from emotional and nervous disorders [12, 13]. Coronary heart disease is now considered pandemic in industrialized, developed societies.

This can be explained if one believes that all health-illness matters have psychological as well as biological components. A comprehensive review of the literature on heart disease shows that there are specific categories of social psychological factors that are related to an increased risk of heart disease. They included intergenerational mobility, incongruity of status, high levels of anxiety, environmental stress, and Type A personalities [13].

Disturbances of the respiratory and circulatory systems are reinforced by the social acceptability of such illnesses. Asthma and heart disease, along with some other disorders (e.g., ulcer) have been reported to be more socially acceptable than disorders such as tuberculosis, carcinoma, and mental illness [25].

Heart-lung conditions that are associated with the ventilation need have many etiological associations. Asthma is a classic example of a disease whose causation is complex. It is associated with many factors: extrinsic factors, such as antigens, dust, and molds, and intrinsic factors, such as chemical substances, bacterial protein, and psychological (affective) factors.

Numerous studies and hypnotic demonstrations have shown that attacks of asthma can be brought on in the absence of allergens by suggesting that an allergen is present. Conversely, if an allergen is present, an asthma attack can be prevented by the hypnotic suggestion that it is absent.

Researchers have further found that "pent-up emotional tension" accompanied by anoxemia occurs in asthma patients and that it can be overcome by motor expressions of emotion, such as "weeping, laughing, acting out of anger, confession, or by an asthma attack" [14].

In studies of the asthma patient, a wide range of techniques has been used, including clinical, pathological, radiological, spectroscopic, oximetric, and psychotherapeutic techniques. Common conclusions have been reached regarding the association of feelings, the rate of inspiration-expiration, and the depth of inspiration-expiration and respiratory disorders. The association has also been demonstrated in persons undergoing grief reactions — grief and grieving are commonly associated with sighing respirations.

In helping with the complex ventilation need in the practice of caring, the nurse must attend to more than the biophysical functions, such as the heart rate, blood chemistries, respiratory rate, and oxygen supply. The meaning and concept of the ventilation need must be broadened if the goal is health care.

The work of Friedman and Rosenman [11] has substantiated some critical aspects of the psychophysiological factors of heart disease. The factors are found in Type A personalities: That is, persons who are excessively punctual, competitive, aggressive, and hostile are more likely than others to suffer from heart disease.

Thus all human needs must be viewed within a context that includes a person's social condition, internal perceptions, methods of coping, and patterns of living, as well as the physical diagnosis of illness.

A striking example of the limitations of health professionals is pointed out by Friedman and Rosenman [11]. They described an incident in which an upholsterer was repairing the chairs in the waiting room of a group of doctors. After the upholsterer had looked at the chairs, he asked the doctors what sort of practice they had. The doctors said that they were cardiologists, and they asked the upholsterer why he wanted to know. The upholsterer replied, "I was just wondering, because it's so peculiar that only the front edges of your chair seats are worn out." The incident indicates a strong behavior pattern of coronary patients; that is, the Type A attributes of tension and impatience are manifested by sitting on the edge of the seat while waiting for the doctor.

Evidence now shows that neither high cholesterol levels nor diets high in fat can explain the incidence of heart disease. Some studies show that the incidence of heart disease in people with the Type A personality is seven times higher than it is in people with the Type B personality. A person with a Type B personality has no sense of the urgency of time, no excessively competitive drive, and no free-floating hostility [11]. The same studies also indicated that a person's serum cholesterol level may be determined as much by the person's feelings as by what he has eaten.

Feelings and stress affect both the lungs and the heart. Feelings and stress strongly affect the gratification of the ventilation need. The use of the respiratory and circulatory systems to handle emotional states seems to be a key element in health maintenance and the treatment of heart-lung diseases. A number of physiological activities are regulated by the ventilation system. The delivery of oxygen to the cells depends on the coordination of the respiratory and circulatory systems. The acts of breathing, modification of breathing during swallowing, coughing, and sneezing, the rate and depth of respiration, the rate of circulation in relation to respiration function are all regulated by the autonomic nervous system, and they affect the ventilation need. The integration and coordination of the respiratory and circulatory systems have to be in relation to all the needs of the person.

A high priority in nursing care is ensuring that the patient always has enough oxygen and that the respiratory and circulatory systems are coordinated to deliver oxygen to the cells. However, to gratify ventilation needs, biophysical care alone is inadequate. The practice of caring that includes assistance with the preventive components of the ventilation need must use a broad, holistic focus that includes ventilation of feelings and thoughts, as well as of the lungs and the rest of the body. The efficiency of the respiratory and circulatory systems is often determined by emotions. The ventilation need is affected by the ventilation (or lack of ventilation) of feelings. For example, anxiety alters the rate and depth of respiration. Irregular respiration occurs during crying. Rapid and shallow respiration occurs in sighing or when a person feels guilt, anger, or resentment. The pulse and heart rates increase with anxiety and fear.

Psychological and organic causes of various respiratory and cardiac conditions are often reported. Studies have shown that esophageal spasms and bronchial widening occur with pleasant suggestions and that bronchial narrowing occurs with unpleasant suggestions. Hyperventilation results in a state of alkalosis in the blood and an increase in carbon dioxide, along with dizziness, muscle tension, pain, and an increased heart rate. Startling or shock causes a momentary cessation of respiration, followed by irregularity in the rhythm and depth of respiration. Stress in general has been reported to give rise

to increases or decreases in the respiratory rate. Stress has
different effects on tidal air volume, and it frequently results
in shallow breathing.

The ventilation of feelings associated with the respiratory
and circulatory systems is a much broader way to view and
understand the ventilation need. Such a view is more consistent with the practice of health prevention than with the
practice of curing.

Caring for the person, as opposed to trying to cure a heart-
lung disorder, necessitates an understanding of the psychosocial variables and feeling states underlying the basic need
and the illness.

The following observations on feelings states and respiratory functioning have been made [28]:

1. An increased rate and(or) depth of respiration and sighing
   are reported to occur with anxiety and sometimes with
   anger and resentment. A decreased rate and(or) depth of
   respiration occur when patients feel tense because of
   anxiety or anger, or when they feel sad or dejected.
2. Irregular respiration has often been associated with anger,
   particularly suppressed anger. Irregular respiration has
   also been associated with guilt and sadness.

Although it may be obvious from numerous studies and the
common experiences of everyone, it should be emphasized
that a healthy release of emotions is related to the ventilation
need, which in turn can affect the respiratory and circulatory
systems. Just as oxygen and blood supplies are necessary for
survival, the ventilation of feelings appears to be necessary for
health maintenance and control of emotional tension. Those
two processes, ventilation of feelings and ventilation of oxygen, are necessary for one's health and well-being. If ventilation of feelings is not provided for, the respiratory and
circulatory systems can be impaired, resulting in heart-lung
diseases and other illnesses.

The need to ventilate feelings can affect not only individuals
but also a whole society. It is interesting to note how individuals, cultural groups, and whole societies channel feelings.

Are feelings of frustration, anger, and aggression ventilated directly and verbally through functional patterns of communication, or is the repression or suppression of feelings encouraged? Are pent-up feelings released destructively through physical violence, riots, crime, assaults, or murders, or through illnesses, especially respiratory or cardiac illnesses? Even though the questions are purely speculative, they are directly associated with health of people and societies.

The health professional should know about the strong link between the need to ventilate emotions and the biophysical ventilation need, which affects respiration and circulation.

The carative factor assistance with the ventilation need can be examined considering the needs of individuals, cultural groups and societies (i.e., the degree to which individuals, cultural groups, and societies allow for the expression of their feelings). It is especially important that the need be examined considering one's role as a health professional. Are the feelings of the nurse or of the patient ignored, denied, blocked, encouraged, or expressed? If they are expressed, how are they expressed? Through direct communication or actions? Constructively or destructively? Or physically, through a system or need?

Psychiatrists and social scientists have suggested that people in the United States have trouble expressing anger. Social restraints in the United States used to be related to inhibition of the expression of sexual feelings, (e.g., the restraints of the Protestant ethic). However, now the questions are, how does U.S. society handle anger or allow for its ventilation? How do families promote or inhibit the expression of anger within the family group — between parents, and between children and parents? Can anger be expressed directly and constructively to promote problem solving and healthy communication? Or is anger inhibited and suppressed and then expressed physically, explosively, or destructively? Are feelings denied, repressed, and then manifested through changes in a biophysical system? Do affective states in turn create problems for the nurse who is trying to help gratify the ventilation need, which extend beyond its overt, tangible aspects?

Some difficulties in the expression of emotions are related

to the expression of anger. People react to anger in three
ways [24] :

1. *Extrapunitively:* by directing anger and hostility onto
   objects or other people in an attempt to handle frustration.
2. *Intropunitively:* by placing anger and hostility onto oneself. Such an approach to anger usually results in blaming
   oneself, low self-esteem, depression, or psychosomatic
   reactions.
3. *Impunitively:* by seeking to neutralize or minimize the
   anger or hostile-aggressive feelings. Such an approach to
   anger is comparable to avoidance or denial. The person
   who uses that approach tries to forget an angry episode or
   not take it seriously. The approach may result in biophysical changes in a bodily system if it becomes one's habitual
   response to anger.

Each of those methods of dealing with anger is appropriate,
realistic, and even common in certain situations. The methods
do not allow direct, functional, verbal expression of anger as a
constructive outlet (e.g., "I feel angry"). When the anger is
difficult to pinpoint or channel directly, constructive physical
outlets can be useful (e.g., engaging in golf, tennis, jogging,
handball, squash, or other physical activities).

Often feelings are not ventilated directly or constructively.
When they are not, intense guilt, fear, and pent-up rage that
manifest themselves in bodily symptoms can result. The circulatory and respiratory systems are likely to be affected in a
person's attempt to gratify his or her ventilation need.

In the practice of caring, the nurse must observe the emotions that need to be released or channeled. That is especially
important in disorders of the ventilatory system. Often emotional stresses aggravate a person's illness.

The nurse also needs to assess her or his own feelings and
how they are channeled or ventilated. In addition, the nurse
must analyze his or her feelings about caring for patients that
have disorders that are characterized by attacks; for example,
asthma, emphysema, and coronary disease. Often patients
with disorders of the ventilatory system need constant

observation, protection, and support. The nurse who knows about the holistic perspective of helping to gratify the ventilation need can better help a patient. Assistance with the ventilation need involves much more than the administration, regulation, or monitoring of oxygen, vital signs, blood pressure, breathing exercises, and medication regimens. The need to ventilate — in the complete sense of the word — involves more than the intake and output of oxygen and carbon dioxide; it encompasses the ventilation of positive and negative feelings — by laughing or crying while expressing joy, sorrow, anger, or frustration. In every instance the result of emotional ventilation is a sense of restoration of the mind, body, and soul. The practice of the science of caring includes a complete perspective of how a person uses his or her ventilatory system not only for breathing but also for coping with feelings and emotions that need an outlet. To help gratify the need to restore one's mind, body, and soul through ventilating one's feelings, the nurse must appreciate the ventilation need and the complex interrelationship of body and mind — between one's bodily systems and one's internal perceptions.

The practice of caring must adopt a humanistic-scientific orientation toward human needs that considers social conditions, patterns of living, and emotions, as well as respiratory-circulatory data. Such a holistic perspective for intervention with the gratification of human needs provides a broad psychosocial, psychosomatic, and cultural focus. High-quality health care includes more than care for only the biophysical need.

Significance of the Ventilation Need for the Practice of Caring

1. The ventilation need includes (1) the respiratory and circulatory systems, (2) the psychological need to ventilate feelings, and (3) the sociocultural norms for releasing emotions.
2. A holistic perspective is useful for viewing a person's ventilation need and understanding his or her health.

3. Specific categories of social and psychological factors have been found to be related to an increased risk of diseases associated with the ventilatory need; for example, heart-lung disease seems to be associated with intergenerational mobility, high levels of anxiety, environmental stress, and the Type A personality.
4. The practice of caring necessitates viewing the ventilation need within a context that includes a person's sociocultural norms, ways of coping, and patterns of living, as well as the demands on his or her biophysical systems.
5. Stress and emotions strongly affect the gratification of the ventilation need. The use of the cardiac and respiratory biophysical-bodily system to handle emotions and feelings is a key element in maintaining health and treating heart-lung diseases.
6. The practice of caring includes concern for the ventilation of the patient's thoughts and feelings as well as for the delivery of oxygen to the lungs and the rest of the body.
7. Just as oxygen and blood are necessary for survival, the need to ventilate feelings is also necessary for health maintenance.
8. If the nurse does not help a patient ventilate his or her feelings, the patient may not ventilate them. If the patient's feelings are not ventilated, his or her prolonged frustration may lead to diseases (especially diseases of the heart or lungs).
9. Although the day-to-day patterns of healthy communication and opportunities for emotional release affect all aspects of health care, they have been found to affect the ventilation need in specific ways.
10. The practice of caring adopts a holistic orientation in understanding the need for ventilation that includes personal, social, and cultural conditions, patterns of living, emotional expression, and respiratory-circulatory functions.

REFERENCES

1. Alexander, F. Fundamental concepts of psychosomatic research. *Psychosomatic Medicine* 3:205, 1943.

2. Alexander, F. Treatment of a case of peptic ulcer and personality disorder. *Psychosomatic Medicine* 9:321, 1947.
3. Alexander, F., and French, T. M. *Psychoanalytic Therapy*. New York: Ronald, 1946.
4. Beland, I. *Clinical Nursing* (2nd ed.). New York: Macmillan, 1970.
5. Bowlby, J. *Attachment*. Attachment and Loss, vol. I. New York: Basic Books, 1969. P. 178.
6. Cannon, W. B. The influence of emotional states on the functions of the alimentary canal. *American Journal of Medical Science* 137:480, 1909.
7. Cannon, W. B. Recent studies of bodily effects of fear, rage, and pain. *Journal of Philosophy, Psychology and Scientific Methods* 11:162, 1914.
8. Cannon, W. B. *The Wisdom of the Body*. New York: Norton, 1932.
9. Cannon, W. B. *Bodily Changes in Pain, Hunger, Fear, and Rage*. New York: Appleton-Century-Crofts, 1939.
10. Carnow, B. W., et al. The role of air pollution in chronic obstructive pulmonary disease. *Journal of the American Medical Association* 214:894, 1970.
11. Friedman, M., and Rosenman, R. H. *Type A Behavior and Your Heart*. New York: Knopf, 1974.
12. Gardner, E. Emotional disorders in medical practice. *Annals of Internal Medicine* 73:651, 1970.
13. Jenkins, D. Psychologic and social precursors of coronary disease, Part I. *New England Journal of Medicine* 284:244, 1971.
14. Lovett Doust, J. W., and Leigh, D. Studies on the physiology of awareness: The interrelationships of emotions, life situations, and anoxemia in patients with bronchial asthma. *Psychosomatic Medicine* 15:292, 1953.
15. Mahl, G. T., and Brody, E. B. Chronic anxiety, symptomatology, experimental stress and HCL secretion. *Archives of Neurology and Psychiatry* 71:314, 1954.
16. Mason, R. E. *Internal Perception and Bodily Functioning*. New York: International Universities Press, 1961.
17. Mayer, J. Obesity control. *American Journal of Nursing* 65:112, 1965.
18. Mayer, J. Some aspects of the problem of regulation of food intake and obesity, Part 1. *New England Journal of Medicine* 274:610, 1966.
19. Mead, M. Cultural Patterns and Technical Change. In I. Beland, *Clinical Nursing*. New York: Macmillan, 1970.
20. Miller, C. A. Current understanding of eating and dieting. *Psychosomatics* 5:119, 1964.
21. Mitchell, P. H. *Concepts Basic to Nursing*. New York: McGraw-Hill, 1973.

22. Murray, R., and Zentner, J. *Nursing Concepts for Health Promotion.* Englewood Cliffs, N.J.: Prentice-Hall, 1975.
23. Plutchik, R. *The Emotions: Facts, Theories and a New Model.* New York: Random House, 1962.
24. Rosenzweig, S. Types of reactions to frustration. *Journal of Abnormal and Social Psychology* 29:298, 1934.
25. Schwab, J. J., Fenneli, E. B., and Warheit, G. J. The epidemiology of psychosomatic disorders. *Psychosomatics* 15;88, 1974.
26. Schwartz, L., and Schwartz, J. *The Psychodynamics of Patient Care.* Englewood Cliffs, N.J.: Prentice-Hall, 1972. P. 63.
27. Solomon, P., and Patch, V. D. (eds.). *Handbook of Psychiatry.* Los Altos, Calif.: Lange, 1974.
28. Stevenson, I. P., and Ripley, H. S. Variations in respiration and respiratory systems during changes in emotions. *Psychosomatic Medicine* 14:476, 1952.
29. Stunkard, A. J. Physical activity, emotions and human obesity. *Psychosomatic Medicine* 20:366, 1958.
30. Sullivan, A. J., and McKell, T. E. *Personality in Peptic Ulcer.* Springfield, Ill.: Thomas, 1950.
31. Tringo, J. The handicapped as a minority. *Human Behavior* 1:127, 1972.
32. Wolf, S. J. Summary of evidence relating life situation and emotional response to peptic ulcer. *Annals of Internal Medicine* 31:637, 1949.
33. Wolf, S. J., and Wolff, H. G. Genesis of peptic ulcer in man. *Journal of the American Medical Association* 120:670, 1942.
34. Wolf, S. J., and Wolff, H. G. Life situation and gastric function: A summary. *American Practitioner* 3:1, 1948.
35. Wolff, H. G. Life stress and bodily disease — A formulation. *Proceedings of the Association for Research in Nervous and Mental Disease* 29:1059, 1949.
36. Wolff, H. G., Grace, W., and Wolf, S. Life situations, emotions, and the large bowel. *Transactions of the Association of American Physicians* 62:192, 1949.

7. ASSISTANCE WITH THE GRATIFICATION OF THE LOWER ORDER PSYCHOPHYSICAL NEEDS

THE ACTIVITY-INACTIVITY NEED

The basic purpose of all human action is the protection, the maintenance, and the enhancement not only of the self but also of the self-concept [27].

A person's need for activity-inactivity is fundamental and central in his or her life. A person's ability to move about and interact with his or her environment gives him or her control over external forces. In addition, the activity-inactivity need is critical in meeting other needs. One's activity need determines one's ability to move about freely and to express one's self. Motion and activity are channels for expressing a range of emotions and exhibiting a range of behaviors and life-styles. Nonverbal communications, such as gestures and facial expressions, are related to the activity need, and they discharge emotions and communicate messages to the environment.

Activity-inactivity serves to channel energy constructively. Activity provides maturation, novelty, mastery, competence, and variety. Forms of inactivity (e.g., relaxation, rest, sleep, reading, and meditation) recharge one's store of energy. Both dimensions of that need are necessary — an expenditure of energy in activities and appropriate, worthwhile ways to replenish energy by forms of inactivity.

One's activity-inactivity level is a vital factor in achieving a balance between one's energy level and the environment. The activity-inactivity need maintains a balance between its two parts (activity = energy expenditure; inactivity = restoration of energy). Both parts are necessary to maintain a balance and to gratify the activity-inactivity need.

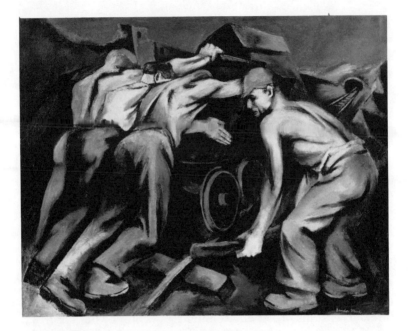

Mine Workers, by Bendor Mark. (Collection, The Denver Art Museum)

The Activity Dimension

The two dimensions of the activity-inactivity need exist on a continuum of energy utilization. Two factors affect the utilization of energy: (1) the expenditure of energy in various activities and (2) a person's tolerance for activity [15]. Whenever a person experiences health-illness changes, his or her activity-inactivity level is affected. The person's adaptations to those changes are major concerns for the nurse who cares for the sick, restores health, or promotes healthy levels of activity-inactivity. A nurse is often in a caring situation in which changes in the person's activity-inactivity levels can be observed. Major interventions related to the activity-inactivity need are within the nurse's territory. Alterations in meeting the need affect the person's coping and need gratification. Likewise, alterations in any of the other human needs affect the gratification of the activity-inactivity need.

Whenever a person is hospitalized there are changes in his or her activity-inactivity level. When a person is weak, his or her tolerance for activity is altered. Even though the person's previous tolerance for an activity may have been high, the same activity in the hospital may require *more* energy. Even so-called healthy persons have different levels of tolerance for activity. An athlete who works out daily has a tolerance that is higher than that of a sedentary office worker who drives to and from work and plays golf on the weekends. If the athlete and the office worker were to participate in the same activity, the sedentary office worker would expend more energy. The phenomenon is illustrated by the "healthy" but sedentary person who has a heart attack after shoveling snow because he has expended more energy than his body could put out. Such an outcome is related to the factors involved with energy utilization and the concept of the activity-inactivity need. A person's tolerance for activity and the amount of energy expended affect a person's healthy gratification of the activity-inactivity need.

Often there is a disagreement between the patient and the health professional about the extent of the change in activity that is necessary to maintain or promote health. Both adults and children maintain their usual activity levels even when health professionals suggest that they do otherwise. A patient with chronic hypertension and coronary heart disease who insists on playing a vigorous game of tennis and continues to ski probably believes that his or her condition is less serious than diagnosed. Engaging in activity is often a sign that one is like "other people" and does not need to limit his or her activity. Frequently, adults and children go to extremes to demonstrate to themselves and others that they are normal.

The nurse's determination of activity levels must include each person's present condition (tolerance level), any demands on the body's energy, and the expenditure of energy required by an activity.

Changes in activity levels can range from overwork and hyperactivity to nonconstructive or immobilized states. Activity levels can be changed in three ways [20]: (1) by disease or trauma, (2) by external restriction through prescribed treatment (e.g., bed rest or mechanical devices), and (3) most commonly, by voluntary curtailment to conserve energy, assist with coping, or to maintain an equilibrium between the external and internal environments.

Other important aspects of the activity-inactivity need are the constructive and nonconstructive features of both of its parts. The constructive aspects of activity include mobility and the tasks of daily living (e.g., getting up, going to work, playing, and developing competence or mastery). These activities promote balance and self-regulation. Constructive releases of energy help to define a person and determine ways in which his or her health and physical fitness are measured. Many people define physical fitness or health in terms of mobility and daily activities [20].

While excessive activity in the face of an obvious need for restraint is a problem for some people, many others are daily affected by the activity need when they seek ways to channel their energy constructively. One of contemporary society's biggest problems is how to use energy in recreation, relaxation, and leisure time. The tendency in the United States is to turn hobbies and relaxing activities into compulsions. On the one hand, leisure activities, sports and recreational events, may become work; on the other hand, people may become passive, inactive spectators (e.g., watchers of TV, movies, and spectator sports; riders instead of walkers). Extreme activity or inactivity can lead to anxiety and guilt about the constructiveness of one's activities. A person may feel guilty when playing; a person may also feel that he or she should be playing instead of doing work.

Too little or too much activity can be unhealthy, and either condition tends to perpetuate itself if it is not interrupted. Scholars who have studied the use of leisure time think that people who are active in their work also tend to be active in their play. People with inactive jobs are usually inactive during leisure activities; they spend time lounging, watching TV, playing cards, reading, napping, and so on.

Marshall McLuhan has discussed the passivity encouraged by TV and commercials [19]. The message of the media is that all one has to do to be active is to buy something ("Join the Pepsi generation").

Different cultures and different eras have used various ways to channel energy constructively. Simpler societies and rural communities today seem to be more successful in channeling energy constructively by providing communal leisure activities (e.g., community events, church activities, bingo, card games, picnics, and club activities).

Some cultural groups and nations have traditional, sanctioned leisure activities (e.g., the fiestas in South America, Mexico, Spain, and southern Europe). Some aboriginal groups have tribal ceremonies. Earlier in its history, the United States had frequent rodeos, revival meetings, hunts, and political gatherings that included the whole community.

Society's failure to provide meaningful activities that are socially acceptable may account for social problems such as violence, delinquency, and disengagement. McLuhan says that society's failure has produced social apathy, anxiety, and alienation. According to McLuhan, society must recognize the subtle effect that TV and passive involvement in activities have on the perceptions and attitudes of children. The child today grows up in a "mythic" world of electronically transmitted data and experiences that are taken for granted. However, the person cannot find a way to involve himself or herself or to discover how he or she relates to the world [19].

However, persons who are socially isolated (e.g., by being confined to bed or prison) or who experience sensory isolation or deprivation often find emotional meaning in certain objects that help channel their energy. Objects serve as a means of action for persons who seek to gratify their activity need. The choice of objects depends on the culture, the era, the situation, and the individual. That is evident in the use that creative people make of objects (e.g., some people who are paralyzed from the neck down do art work with their mouth and teeth; some people in prison train birds). The use one makes of objects depends on three things:

1. The possibilities for action that the person perceives in the object
2. One's general readiness to do the kind of action suggested by an object
3. One's state at the moment

Those three components influence what action is taken by someone who has major inhibitions about gratifying his or her activity need because of illness, isolation, or deprivation. Objects that are usually considered meaningless or are ignored by a person become very important when emotional meanings and possibilities for action develop or emerge for the person. A person confined to a hospital for a long time seeks to use objects in the hospital as meaningful outlets for his or her energy. The nurse can help with that.

An arthritic elderly person whose satisfaction throughout life has come from building cabinets may need to change his or her previous activity (and previous objects of action). A change in one's activity level necessitates a change in perception of the body's tolerance for activity as well as a change in perception of objects that can be used in action. For example, the arthritic cabinet maker may begin to see possibilities for action in pieces of wood that could be used for works of art. Before the change in his or her activity level, the cabinet maker saw only the cabinet-making possibilities of wood. If one changes to accommodate the change in one's activity level, objects take on different meanings for action. Thus the caring person can help another to perceive himself or herself accurately and to develop his or her higher order needs. Direct gratification of one's needs also promotes achievement and possibly even self-actualization. The practice of caring should attempt to identify and develop the resources of each person to assist in the gratification of the activity need.

Human beings are unique in their ability and need to control important features of their environment. Depending on the intensity and circumstances of the activity need, there is usually an urge to find out about any change in one's environment and to test the effects of one's action on it. A dramatic example of that urge is Benjamin Franklin's experiment with a kite in a thunderstorm. Other less widely-known events are equally dramatic (the taming and training of birds by the "Birdman of Alcatraz"; the art work of the paralyzed girl who used her teeth and mouth to move her pen). Those examples suggest the need for not only activity but also novelty, competence, and achievement, which are usually dependent on mobility.

Constructive forms of activity-inactivity are essential for people's biological, psychological, and sociocultural functioning. Biological activity is necessary to maintain strength, endurance, and coordination of the muscles. It promotes internal physiological processes at the cellular level through metabolism, cellular nutrition, and the blood's circulation. Activity at the cellular level provides outlets for constructive energy for all the bodily systems [20]. It is generally acknowledged by professionals and the public that bed rest can be detrimental to one's physical functioning; out-of-bed activity keeps muscles in tone and supports the body's muscular and skeletal systems. Lung capacity, circulatory capacity, and physical tolerance are all determined or affected by activities and in turn affect the body's functioning.

Constructive activities of daily life are important aspects of development because they teach the methods and pleasures of accomplishment, mastery, and control of one's environment. One's self-concept, self-esteem and self-worth are affected by how successfully one channels one's energy through constructive activities. When one's activity level is altered, independence, self-concept, self-esteem, and self-worth are affected. The psychological effects of a change in one's activity level can often be subtle, and they may be overlooked by the nurse. The nurse must be attentive to the psychological effects of altered activities from both subjective and objective perspectives. To better appreciate the subtle psychology of the experience that a change in activity brings, the following selection from *Psychology of the Sickbed** is included. The changes in activity described here were caused by a mild illness. How much more important the psychological experience must be for the person who has a progressive or permanent change in activity!

After a restless and disturbed sleep, I wake up in the morning, not feeling too well. I get out of bed, however, intending to start the day in the usual manner. But soon I notice that I cannot. I have a headache; I feel sick. I notice an uncontrollable urge to vomit and I deem myself so incapable of facing the day that I convince myself that I am ill. I return

*Reprinted from *Psychology of the Sickbed* by J. H. van den Berg by permission of Duquesne University Press.

to the bed I just left with every intention of staying there for a while. The thermometer shows that my decision was not unreasonable. My wife's cautious inquiry whether I would like something for breakfast makes the reason much clearer. I am *really* ill. I give up my coffee and toast, as I give up everything the day was to bring, all the plans and the duties. And to prove that I am abandoning these completely I turn to the wall, nestle myself in my bed, which guarantees a comparative well-being by its warm invitation to passivity, and close my eyes. But I find that I cannot sleep.

Then, slowly, but surely, a change, characteristic of the sickbed, establishes itself. I hear the day begin. From downstairs the sounds of the household activities penetrate into the bedroom. The children are called for breakfast. Loud hasty voices are evidence of the fact that their owners have to go to school in a few minutes. A handkerchief has to be found, and a bookbag. Quick young legs run up and down the stairs. How familiar, and at the same time how utterly strange things are; how near and yet how far away they are. What I am hearing is the beginning of my daily existence, with this difference, though, that now I have no function in it. In a way I still belong completely to what happens downstairs; I take a share in the noises I hear, but at the same time everything passes me by, everything happens at a great distance. "Is Daddy ill?" a voice calls out; even at this early moment, it has ceased to consider that I can hear it. "Yes, Daddy is ill." A moment later the door opens and they come to say goodbye. They remain just as remote. The distance I measured in the sounds from downstairs appears even greater, if possible, now that they are at my bedside, with their fresh clean faces and lively gestures. Everything about them indicates the normal healthy day, the day of work and play, of street and school. The day outside the house, in which "outside" has acquired a new special meaning for me, a meaning emphasizing my exclusion.

I hear that the day has begun out in the street. It makes itself heard; cars pull away and blow their horns; and boys shout to one another. I have not heard the sound of the street like this for years, from such an enormous distance. The doorbell rings; it is the milkman, the postman, or an acquaintance; whoever it is I have nothing to do with him. The telephone rings; for a moment I try to be interested enough to listen, but again I soon submit to the inevitable, reassuring, but at the same time slightly discouraging, knowledge that I have to relinquish everything. I have ceased to belong; I have no part in it.

The world has shrunk to the size of my bedroom, or rather my bed. For even if I set foot on the floor it seems as if I am entering a *terra incognita*. Going to the bathroom is an unfriendly, slightly unreal, excursion. With the feeling of coming home I pull the blankets over me. The horizon is narrowed to the edge of my bed and even this bed is not completely my domain. Apart from where I am lying it is cold and uncomfortable; the pillow only welcomes me where my head touches it. Every move is a small conquest.

CHANGE OF THE FUTURE AND THE PAST

The horizon in time too is narrowed. The plans of yesterday lose their meaning and their importance; they have hardly any real value. They seem more complicated, more exhausting, more foolish and ambitious than I saw them the day before. All that awaits me becomes tasteless, or even distasteful. The past seems saturated with trivialities. It appears to me that I hardly ever tackled my real tasks. Future and past lose their outlines; I withdraw from both and I live in the confined present of this bed which guards me against the things that were and those that will be. Under normal circumstances I live in the future, and in the past as far as the future draws upon it to prescribe my duties. Apart from a few special moments I never really live in the present, I never think of it. But the sickbed does not allow me to escape from the present.

Normally I am not aware of my body; it performs its tasks like an instrument. Now that I am ill, I become acutely aware of a bodily existence, which makes itself felt in a general malaise, in a dull headache and in a vague nausea. The body which used to be a condition becomes the sole content of the moment. The present, while always serving the future, and therefore often being an effect of the past, becomes saturated with itself. As a patient I live with a useless body in a disconnected present.

Everything gets an "actual" meaning, and this is quite a discovery for us who are pledged to the future. The telephone, rather than conveying the message from the person at the other end of the line, makes me aware of the fact that, as a frozen appeal, it rings with a new sound through a house which has become remarkably remote and strange. The blankets of my bed, articles so much devoted to utility that they used to disappear behind the goal they served, so that in my normal condition I could not possibly have said what color they are, become jungles of colored threads in which my eye laboriously finds its way. The sheets are immeasurable white plains with deep crevasses, steep slopes and insurmountable summits; a polar landscape to the paralyzed traveller that I am.

The wallpaper which I only noticed vaguely, if I ever saw it at all, has to be painfully analyzed in lines, dots, smaller and larger figures. I feel an urge to examine the symmetrical pattern, and to see in it caricatures of people, animals and things. It is as if I am taking a Rorschach test, immensely enlarged. Hopeless and nightmarish interpretations urge themselves upon me, particularly when I am running a fever. And I feel I am going mad when I find a spot that cannot be made to fit into the structure which took me such pains to evolve.

After a few days I begin to hate the oil painting on the wall. For by this time I have acquired a certain freedom to change the caricatures of the wallpaper; I can replace the configuration I created by another one when I am bored with it. But the figures in the painting, the people, the animals, the houses and the trees, resist every attempt in this direction. The hunter, about to shoot the flying duck, remains aiming motionlessly, while I have judged his chances a hundred times. And the duck, which would probably manage to reach a hiding place if it is quick enough, defies all dangers as it comfortably floats over the landscape where the sun forgets the laws of cosmography in an eternal sunset. "Oh! please, hurry up" I say, exasperated, and even if I am amused at my own words, I do ask the next visitor to please be kind enough either to turn the picture to the wall or to remove it altogether.

THE CALL OF THINGS

As I notice my clothes, hanging over the chair at the foot of my bed, I realize with a new clarity that the horizon of my existence is narrowed. For the jacket there, the shirt and tie, belong to the outside world. I see myself descending the stairs, going to work, and receiving guests. Certainly I am that man, but at the same time, I have ceased to be him. The clothes are completely familiar and very near, and yet they belong just as truly to a world which is no longer mine. I feel a vague sympathy for these clothes, which remind me, tactfully, of my healthy existence, which must have had its value. Nevertheless, I am pleased when caring hands change my bedroom into a proper sickroom and my clothes are put away in the wardrobe. For however tactful the reminder is, I do not like to be reminded at all. After all, I cannot and will not put it into effect anyway.

If I am sensitive this way, if I possess the remarkable sense which enables people to understand the language of the lifeless objects, the discovery of my shoes is particularly revealing, even if I find it hard to put into words what these shoes, with their silent and yet expressive faces, have to say. In his famous journal [Journal II, 1935-1939, Plon, Paris, 1939, p. 232], Julian Green drew our attention to the fact that it is the hat and shoes that are the most personal of our clothes. None of our clothes is entirely anonymous; they are all part of ourselves in a way, an extra skin, the skin that we choose to show others and which we want to see ourselves. We choose our various articles of clothing with this showing and seeing in mind.

A man has not very much choice in this respect. A suit is a suit; the colors may vary a bit, the material and the cut may depend on the amount of money he can afford or is willing to spend. But that is all the variety at his disposal. A man who respects himself buys a shirt that hardly differs from the one his neighbor or colleague wears. In the matter of ties we are less restricted. The salesman shows us a rainbow of colors and an array of designs. A tie can be a very personal thing. That is why we are not really pleased to find another man wearing the same tie; it seems as if we meet an attribute of ourselves which he has unlawfully appropriated.

And then the hat. Even for men the varieties in color, shape, consistency, hairiness and handiness are almost inexhaustible. It becomes even more personal when the first newness has worn off. The hat acquires dents and creases; the brim gets a twist and a wave. These things are all signatures of the wearer and show his hold on things, his way of life. There are crying hats, proud hats, provocative hats, gloomy hats, tortured hats. And just as they tell us something about their respective owners, they certainly have something to say to their wearers themselves. Will the owner of the gloomy hat not be touched with a certain pity when he sees his hat hanging among happier members of its kind.

Shoes, too, form a very personal part of our clothing. Besides that, they enjoy the extraordinary privilege of having faces. Some shoes shake with laughter, others stare silently upon a vague distance; others again look at us full of reproach. In a store we cannot see these things yet; in their distinctive neutrality they make our choice difficult. But we have only to wear our new acquisitions a few weeks and the personality is there. As a result their faces are not unlike those of their wardrobe-mates. After all, they are of one family. Our shoes constitute our contact with the earth; they tread on country lanes and city streets. Their route is our life's course. Now they are waiting for us, there, by the bed, a silent but futile invitation. The faces with which they look at me completely explain my condition; I no longer belong to the life which nonetheless is still mine; my street, my road, lies outside the horizon of my existence.

The author of the preceding selection helps the reader appreciate the psychological experience of a person undergoing a change in activity level. A holistic approach is necessary in understanding the need for activity and how it is affected by health change and illness.

Regression occurs, as well as feelings of fear, frustration, loneliness, isolation, and dependency. A change in activity interferes with the ability of a person to meet his or her lower level biophysical needs (the food and fluid need, the elimination need, and the ventilation need). A change in activity level causes one to become dependent on others to gratify his or her lower level needs, and it also interferes with the gratification of one's higher order needs (the achievement, affiliation, and self-actualization needs). A change in activity can interfere with both higher order and lower order needs.

If someone is unable for any reason to gratify his or her activity need, he or she becomes more occupied with gratification of lower level needs. If the lower level needs are not gratified, energy is concentrated on meeting those needs before progressing to gratification of higher order needs. The lower

order needs dominate. Frustration of the lower order needs
is more localized, more tangible, and more limiting than are
frustrations of the higher order needs. The immediate concern
of the person and nurse often is to attempt to gratify the lower
level needs. However, a holistic focus is necessary for quality
health and higher level development.

Holistic aspects of the activity need are often overlooked
during illness, especially such small activity needs as the need
for a shave, a glass of water, having one's teeth brushed, a
mirror, make-up, looking out the window, or a newspaper.
Those are examples of lower order needs that the healthy person takes for granted. If the needs are inhibited by a change
in activity due to altered health, the needs become more dominant, more localized, and more acute.

When specific activity needs are not gratified, the results
are frustration, anger, bitterness, and regression to a lower
order of functioning in an attempt to gain control. Such
frustration of the lower needs in a hospital usually causes
more complaints about the food, nurses, doctors, hospital,
medication, and so on. The patient may appear comfortable
but be experiencing severe internal discomfort due to the inhibition of lower order needs. In the practice of caring, the
nurse must perceive the need and provide the comfort. She
or he must discover how the patient perceives himself or herself and his or her situation.

Anticipating and attending to specific lower order needs
are critical for the practice of caring. Only when the lower
order needs are gratified can the patient's higher order needs
be effectively gratified. The higher order sociocultural functioning is also affected by activity levels. Mobility, independence, mastery, and environmental control help determine
one's role in the culture and in society. Activity ability over-
laps the achievement need (discussed on pp. 175–183). People
who cannot participate in normal activities often suffer social
stigmatization and discrimination. Disabled and deformed
people are subjected to social pressures and exclusion. Energy
expenditure is necessary for maintaining one's self-concept
and self-worth, as is using energy for successful activities.
Activities affect not only one's achievement need but also

one's affiliation and self-actualization needs. The interpersonal relationships associated with work, leisure, and social activities are affected by changes in one's activity level.

As one can see, the activity-inactivity need is a complex one that includes energy expenditure as well as energy replenishment. Just as activity is essential for people's holistic functioning, so is inactivity. Both dimensions are essential for the biological, psychological, and sociocultural functioning of humans.

The Inactivity Dimension
Sleep. The activity dimension was discussed in the preceding paragraphs, and the inactivity dimension will be discussed in the following paragraphs as being equally important. Sleep is considered a constructive form of inactivity.

Even though activity and inactivity exist on a continuum of energy utilization, they have a biorhythmic pattern that is self-sustaining. There are *exogenous rhythms,* which depend on the external environment (e.g., seasonal variations, lunar cycles, night and day cycles) [7]. Exogenous rhythms help people achieve an internal balance with external stimuli. There are also *endogenous rhythms,* which are internal regulations, such as sleep-wake and sleep-dream cycles. The two cycles generally function in harmony, but changes in one cycle affect the other. The changes do not necessarily synchronize.

The internal biorhythm that affects a person's daily (24-hour) cycle is called the circadian cycle or circadian rhythm. The circadian cycle is perhaps the most prominent biorhythm [7, 21]. Hundreds of physiological-psychological cycles have a length of about 24 hours (e.g., body temperature, heart beat, blood pressure, and kidney output). Levels of alertness, fatigue, social patterns, and irritability are also manifested in a rhythmic pattern in humans. Alternation of the waking and sleep states is the most overt pattern of the circadian cycle related to the inactivity need.

Activity occurs during a person's usual period of waking. The waking state provides the greatest opportunity for decision making and physical activity. The sleep state provides the least opportunity for those functions.

The need for inactivity is related to sleep and its function. Inactivity (sleep and rest) helps a person to conserve and replenish energy. It helps to balance the energy expenditure from one's daily activities. Until recently the physical, carative aspect of sleep was emphasized; that is, people believed sleep was a time for the muscles and organs of the body to rest and repair themselves. Recently, the nature of sleep and its functions have been studied scientifically, and new knowledge relevant to the inactivity need is available.

Sleep has been divided into Stages 1, 2, 3, and 4. *Stage 1* sleep still resembles wakefulness as measured by cortical activity, muscle tone, and eye movement. The physiological measurements are obtained by the electroencephalogram (EEG), the electromyogram (EMG), and the electrooculogram (EOG). During Stage 1 sleep the person may be (1) aware of movements, (2) easily awakened, and (3) in a dreamlike state.

Stages 2 and 3 of sleep show a progressive decrease of cortical activity, relaxation of muscles, and slow, rolling movements of the eyes. In *Stage 4* sleep cortical activity is synchronous, muscles are very relaxed, and major eye movements are infrequent.

During a sleep cycle a person progresses in an orderly fashion through those stages. From Stage 1 a person descends into Stages 2 and 3. After progressively deepening sleep, the person enters Stage 4. In Stage 4 the person is unresponsive to most external stimuli. A pattern of transitions between cycles develops throughout the sleep period; that is, after 10 to 30 minutes of Stage 4 sleep, the person returns to Stage 3 and Stage 2. After a return to Stage 2, the person enters a totally different kind of sleep, called *REM (rapid eyeball movement) sleep.* REM sleep is characterized by a quick, synchronized movement of both eyes as measured by the EOG. REM sleep is thought to be the state most distant from waking. In REM sleep the muscles are also profoundly relaxed.

However, in spite of the depth of REM sleep and its muscular relaxation, the brain's activity is increased. It is during REM sleep that people dream. It has been established that everyone dreams even though he or she may not remember the dreams.

Although sleep is considered essential for energy conservation and replenishment, the sleeping state is not passive. It is paradoxical that during sleep the muscles are profoundly relaxed while brain activity is increased, generally with an increase in the vital signs.

The increase in cortical activity and the vital signs is associated with dreaming even though the function of dreaming is unknown. It seems as though the biophysical replenishment results from the muscular relaxation, whereas the psychological replenishment somehow results from the cortical activity that accompanies dreaming. Of course there are various theories to explain dreams and their role in behavior and psychological functioning. In a psychodynamic interpretation, a dream may help a person rework or resolve psychological conflicts or repressed associations resulting from the mental activities of the day. Some researchers suggest that REM sleep provides a cognitive processing of the recorded data of recent sensory experiences or that it establishes new neural pathways for storing and retrieving data [7, 21]. Others hypothesize that dreaming during REM sleep prepares the person to meet stress when awake and that it may relate to coping mechanisms.

Sleep deprivation studies further validate the mentally restorative function of dreams. People often feel irritable and mildly depressed after only one night of reduced sleep. With sleep deprivation, performance generally declines, and with several days of sleep deprivation the person may experience delusions or hallucinations or become confused and apathetic. As one can see, the effects of sleep deprivation are psychological rather than physiological. Interestingly, when a person is permitted to sleep after deprivation most of the sleep is Stage 4 and REM sleep.

REM sleep is considered unique. Even though its function is unknown, it is closely associated with mental and psychological processes, and it is considered vital to the gratification of the activity-inactivity need.

The inactivity dimension of the need is especially relevant to nursing as the science of caring. Altered states of sleep are common health problems. Hospitalization and treatment regimens contribute to sleep deprivation or a nonconstructive use of sleep. The circadian cycle is frequently upset when one is ill, receiving treatment, or hospitalized.

The use of sleeping pills is related to the inactivity dimension of sleep. The effects of such drugs on sleep — and REM sleep in particular — are relevant to nursing and contribute to the knowledge needed for the knowledge of caring.

Research on sleep has substantiated that most hypnotic drugs that affect the central nervous system affect the quality of sleep, especially REM sleep. It has been established that hypnotic drugs reduce one's normal REM sleeping time up to about two weeks. After a person stops using hypnotics, he or she experiences a rise in REM sleep (40 percent), as contrasted with other types of sleep (25 percent) [7]. The increase in REM sleep may last five weeks or longer after only two weeks of using hypnotics. The rise in REM sleep is frequently accompanied by nightmares, vivid dreams, and a fatigued feeling on awakening.

Besides hypnotic drugs, amphetamines, alcohol, antidepressants, tranquilizers, and opiates may also cause a reduction in REM sleep.

The fact that the body needs to "make up" REM sleep after both sleep deprivation and the use of medication that affects the central nervous system is significant. It suggests that the quality of sleep, especially sleep related to psychological and cognitive functioning, is affected. Even though the research on the subject is valuable and gives guidance and awareness to nursing intervention, further nursing research is needed. Additional investigation can help nursing to develop a base of scientific knowledge relevant to the carative factor assistance with gratification of the activity-inactivity need.

Rest. Rest is another form of inactivity that can be useful. Rest is a de-accelerated state of physical and mental activity in which there is less energy utilization because there is less energy output and input. During rest, energy is conserved and restored. The way a person perceives and values rest determines how he or she seeks to obtain it. Some persons may consider a nap as an opportunity to rest; others may consider a rest as traveling to another location and engaging in different activities. One's past experiences and usual patterns of activity determine one's idea of rest and its effect on one's behavior. The nurse must appreciate the patient's subjective view of rest, because if the patient does not perceive a situation as restful, the rest in that situation may be nonconstructive. What the nurse considers restful (e.g., hospitalization or bed rest) may be tiring for the patient if the external environment is disruptive and the patient is irritated by the "restful" situation.

Fatigue (nonconstructive activity). A "restful" situation that is not restful for the person involved may result in fatigue. Fatigue is the subjective sense of weariness that results from physical or mental exertion [15]. Even if a person is able to achieve physical rest, fatigue sets in if mental exertion occurs. Prolonged mental and physical activity results in fatigue and impaired efficiency.

If fatigue is acute, recovery occurs after rest and sleep. If fatigue is progressive or chronic, rest and sleep become difficult, and the person may develop physical and psychosomatic complaints.

When there is a balance of energy utilization and replenishment, fatigue is not a problem. However, in U.S. society fatigue borders on the boredom and frustration related to a lack of constructive channeling of energy. Fatiguing energy outputs such as worry, unhappiness, conflicts, or tension seem to occur more often in a technological, progressive civilization. Many people who seek medical care have vague but numerous complaints of excessive tiredness or lack of energy. Often such tiredness is related to a lack of meaningful activities. Consequently, people become bored, unhappy, and worried, and they use excessive mental energy through anguish rather than through meaningful and fulfilling cognitive or behavioral activities. The nurse often must assist a patient with gratification of the inactivity need. Perhaps in some instances fatigue can be overcome by rechanneling the patient's energy into constructive channels and new activities.

*Significance of the Activity-Inactivity Need
for the Practice of Caring*

1. The activity-inactivity need is a human need that affects all persons and events with which the nurse is involved.
2. The activity-inactivity need channels energy constructively to balance energy utilization and energy replenishment.
3. The activity-inactivity need provides maturation, mastery, competence, variety, relaxation, and restoration.
4. Inhibition of the activity-inactivity need can thwart gratification of the other human needs and cause the lower order needs to dominate.
5. The lower order, more localized, tangible needs must be gratified before one can gratify the higher order needs; therefore, frustration of the lower order needs can inhibit fulfillment of the higher order needs of achievement, affiliation, and self-actualization.
6. Health regimens and(or) treatments of illness frequently necessitate a change in one's activity level. A change in a person's activity level causes acute subjective experiences for the person that can best be understood from the person's point of view.
7. Depending on the person's inhibition, motivation, and other variables, a person may use an experience of social, psychological, and physical isolation to create new activities with objects in his or her environment.
8. The practice of caring includes assistance with channeling energy constructively (e.g., by altering energy outlets for balanced expenditure or decreasing energy inputs for replenishment).
9. The inactivity necessary for energy replenishment includes constructive forms of inactivity (e.g., rest and sleep). Fatigue and boredom are examples of nonconstructive forms of inactivity.
10. Sleep research has important implications for nursing as the science of caring. Knowledge of the circadian cycle, sleep cycle and REM sleep pattern can be very helpful in assisting with gratification of the activity-inactivity need.

11. Knowledge of the effects of drugs and sleep deprivation on sleep and dreaming is valuable for planning, implementing, and evaluating nursing care.
12. Activity and inactivity should be considered vital aspects of one's biophysical, psychological, and sociocultural well-being.
13. Nursing can become the science of caring by utilizing the available knowledge of the activity-inactivity need and continuing research on the nature, function, and relationship of activity-inactivity to people's health and well-being.

THE SEXUALITY NEED

Sexual satisfaction and fulfillment depend upon the degree to which a man has confidence and pleasure in his masculinity and a woman has satisfaction and pleasure in her femininity and the degree to which both a man and woman have given up childhood attachments to parents and possess means of completely loving another [11].

The sexuality need involves one's complete personality development, including one's sexual identification, self-concept, self-esteem, and related patterns of behavior. The sexuality need is not limited to sexual-genital intercourse; it involves satisfaction with one's body and one's sex and good attitudes toward one's own sex and sexual role. Sometimes the term sexuality is distinguished from the term sexual, sexuality referring to all the things that make one male or female and sexual referring to genital sex. In that sense, the sexual (genital) need is influenced primarily by human biology, but it is controlled mostly by psychological, sociocultural mechanisms.

The sexuality need is biological in nature, and it begins with conception-birth.

It is thought that human sexual behavior is acquired, not innate. Sexual behavior is learned behavior rather than instinctual behavior. Chimpanzees who are deprived of the opportunity to learn sexual behavior do not know how to behave sexually at first. The Harlow studies of monkeys indicate that personal contact is necessary for future social interaction. The

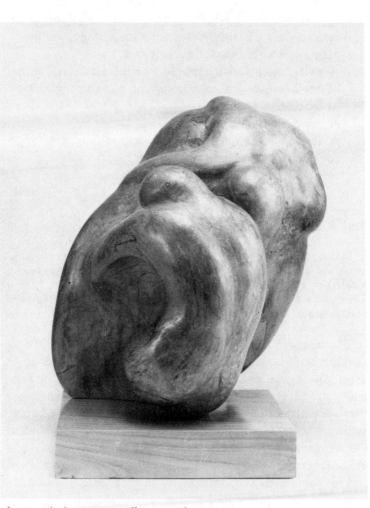

The Couple, by Lipa. (Collection, The Denver Art Museum)

differences between the sexual behaviors of humans and animals are those of degree and kind. The higher an animal is on
the phylogenetic scale, the more mental its sexual behavior is —
and the less biologically controlled.

The early parent-child attachment and trust relationship lays
the foundation for the psychological development of the sexuality need, which is related to sucking, biting, and feeding,
as well as to contact and security. The sexuality need becomes

more developed during the child's preschool years. Freud used the term oedipal stage to describe the early developmental stage of sexual identification and attitude formation about one's sexuality and all that entails. During that stage, sexual curiosity, exploration, imitative dramatic play, and masturbation are common and normal.

Erikson feels that the early establishment of one's sexuality is manifested in the psychological conflict between "initiative versus guilt."

During the adolescent stage of development, the person is struggling with complex genital sexual development and with other physical and psychological changes. Accompanying those changes are new relationships between the sexes. Adolescents need to understand the changes occurring in their bodies, and they may need information about reproduction. They often need help in dealing with their feelings and attitudes about those changes. Adolescence is also a time of struggle in regard to one's identity, sexual role, dating behavior, and future decisions.

The full actualization of sexuality need and biological and psychological maturity culminate during the young adult stage of development. That stage is characterized as a conflict between "intimacy versus isolation," and it is related to the ability to enter into close, meaningful relationships with others. One's ideas about oneself as husband and father or wife and mother are developed. Parenting often brings to a head one's struggle with or resolution of the problems of sexuality. Erikson identified three different reconciliations associated with the sexuality need:

1. The reconciliation of genital orgasm and extragenital sexual needs
2. The reconciliation of love and sexuality
3. The reconciliation of sexual, procreative, and work-productive patterns

In identifying the reconciliations necessary for sexual maturity, Erikson also associates sexuality with the *relationships* of sex and play, of play and work, and of work and sex.

Therefore, one's sexual reconciliations are related to one's life. Maturity includes the ability to regulate the cycles of work, genital sex (procreation), and recreation.

The goals of a mature adult's sexuality include (1) orgasm capacity, (2) with a loved partner, (3) usually one of the opposite sex, and (4) with whom one is able and willing to share a mutual trust and intimacy. Mature sexual development is also related to the ability to procreate and(or) provide a secure environment for one's children [9, 10].

The sexuality need continues to be dominant during old age despite the prevailing myth that sexuality is not a characteristic of old people. The elderly person's sexual activity is largely dependent on the availability of a partner and on his or her own health. An elderly person's sexual need is not necessarily expressed through sexual intercourse; it can also be expressed in the need for continued closeness, affection, and intimacy. Some elderly people continue to have an erotic love interest. Romance is an important part of their sexuality need [24].

The psychosocial interrelationships and reconciliations of one's gender, sexuality, and life in general become more important than the biological aspects of sex. The essence of sexuality is how one relates to other people. In that sense, sexuality is closely linked with affiliative behaviors. Sexuality is related to the total functioning of a person as a man or a woman; it consists of the relationships that a person forms in all his or her daily living experiences, not just in his or her sexual experiences.

In contemporary U.S. society, a wide variety of life-styles can lead to gratification of the sexuality need. One can select marriage or nonmarriage, to have children or not to have children, to live with another person without marriage, to relate to the opposite sex or to the same sex, or to sublimate one's sexual need in work, achievement, service to others, a career, and so on. Despite the wide variety of choices, there are still psychological, social, religious, and moral restraints that affect sexual activities and gratification of the sexuality need. Sexual behavior is affected by guilt, self-concept, fear of inadequacy, or even discrimination. The recent activities of gay coalition groups attest to the social, moral and economic barriers that are erected in the face of nontraditional sexual behavior. Despite the current social openness and frankness regarding sex, society still places expectations and structured norms on sexual behavior.

The sociocultural attitudes toward overt sexual behavior take a variety of forms; the behavior may be encouraged, permitted, condoned, ignored, condemned, or suppressed. Sexual behavior becomes a matter of concern when it violates or is in conflict with cherished social or cultural expectations and values.

The patterns of sexual behavior that exist at any time reflect the degree to which the mores are obeyed or violated. Sexual matters are evaluated and treated quite differently in different societies and different ages. In the words of Shakespeare, "There is nothing either good or bad but thinking makes it so."

In Western culture, the contemporary heterosexual values reflect the two coexisting and conflicting attitudes toward sex. On the one hand, erotic love is portrayed as sinful or wrong. On the other hand, if romantic love is present, erotic love is considered justified. Both attitudes are extreme, and they are incompatible with day-to-day sexual expression.

Because of various value systems and conflicting sociocultural philosophies, male-female sexual activities are highly structured. That fact is demonstrated by the customs of random dating, going steady, being engaged to be engaged, engagement, and, more recently, living together, with patterns of sexual behavior.

In spite of Western society's homogenous rules and sanctions surrounding sexual behavior, there are few universal codes of sexual behavior. The two codes that seem to be universal are:

1. The expectation and right of sexual intercourse between marital partners
2. The prohibition against incestuous relations between parent and child

In addition to those supposedly universal sexual codes, certain other matters related to sexuality are considered universal.
They are impotency, infertility, sexual jealousy, availability
of sexual partners within and outside of marriage, sexual
attractiveness, adultery, and premarital coitus. Those concerns are evaluated and treated quite differently in different
societies and different ages. For example, in some societies
adultery is a sin, in others a violation of property rights, and
in others punishable by death; still other societies allow wives
to have sexual relations with men other than their husbands.
In those societies adultery is not a problem, and there is often
not even a word in the language to identify the act. Again,
the disjunction illustrates that sexual behavior becomes a
matter of concern when it violates or is in conflict cherished
social expectations and values.

What it means to be a woman or a man is a product of at
least three interrelated processes: (1) one's inner (physiological) environment, (2) one's sociocultural environment,
and (3) one's psychological development from birth on [14].
Thus sexual differences or sexual identity is the result of a
complex interaction of internal and external forces in a social
milieu. How those interactions become manifest is determined
by one's individual differences, personality patterns, and developmental experiences. Differing resolutions of developmental
conflicts and differing sexual identification processes further
contribute to what it means to be a woman or a man for an
individual.

Of course, even though a complex interaction determines
one's sexual identity and satisfaction, people grow into male
or female roles along somewhat different paths simply because
they are males or females. Part of one's developing sense of
self relates to being male or to being female. One's society and
culture in turn largely determine the extent to which sexual
differences are emphasized.

Society uses certain stereotypes to portray men and women
as *opposites* [5]. Women are perceived as less competent,
independent, objective, and logical than men; men are perceived as having less interpersonal sensitivity, warmth, and
expressiveness than women. Mental health professionals are

reported to consider mature, healthy women more submissive
and less independent than either mature, healthy men or
adults in general. Thus women are put in a double bind by
the fact that different social standards exist for women than
for adults in general. More important, men and women are
reported to incorporate the positive and negative traits of the
appropriate stereotypes into their self-concepts. "Since more
feminine traits are negatively valued than are masculine traits,
women tend to have more negative self-concepts than do
men" [5].

Through socialization, sexual stereotypes become internalized not only by men and women but also by those in the
health professions. Sexual stereotypes affect one's personality,
and they may also affect the type of care one receives, as well
as the roles that different professions (e.g., medicine and nursing) play in the delivery of health care.

Several important themes have emerged from the data collected on sexual differences and personality. The differences
between men and women are related to *self-esteem, fear of
success, types of motivation,* and *personality traits* [14].

Simone de Beauvoir [3], has written about women's self-
esteem. She described women as having an *object* role and
men as having a *subject* role; thus men are described as active
manipulators who control the world of objects. Women
also are men's objects, and women are manipulated, controlled,
and rendered passive. Women tend to be rewarded for how
they appear to others (as objects), whereas men are rewarded
and valued for what they accomplish (as subjects). Women
have less self-esteem because the sources of self-esteem are
different for men and women, and also because different
expectations, rewards, and values are placed on male and
female accomplishments.

A recent work study [13] shows that more women than
men fear scholastic success. Nine percent of the men studied
feared success, whereas more than 65 percent of the women
studied feared success.

Women often associate excellence with loss of femininity,
social rejection, and personal or societal destruction. A typical
example is that of a woman who deliberately lowers her

academic standing in order to help a male student. A more extreme example is that of the woman who drops out of school to marry and to help her husband complete school while she raises their children [13].

According to the evidence, women cannot easily reconcile success and their feminine identities, whereas men find no discrepancy between success and their masculine identities.

Sexual differences in people's motivation for achievement are mentioned on pages 175–183, but they are discussed in the following paragraphs as related to the sexuality need. As mentioned, the motivation to achieve drives a person to achieve excellence in any field. Motivation is internalized as a personality characteristic. Thus some people have great achievement motivation and others do not.

Several scholars have found that women are more responsive than men to affiliation motives and that men are more responsive than women to achievement motives [12, 26].

It appears that the meaning of achievement is different for men and women. Internal standards of excellence are motives for men, whereas external supports are important motives for women's achievement.

The types of sexual differences discussed in this book emphasize the importance of other factors in understanding sexuality as a gestalt. Sexuality and the fulfillment of one's sexuality affect one's entire personality, sex concept, and social growth and development.

Just as there is research that contributes to the gestalt of sexuality, so also are there irrational and mythical stereotypes about sexuality that contribute equally to one's views of sex and sexuality. Myths and misinformation cloud one's understanding of the human sexuality need (e.g., Alcohol is a sexual stimulant; One must have an orgasm to enjoy sex; Masturbation is harmful; Taking the pill will delay menopause) [8].

Some of society's previously held myths (e.g., Women are not interested in sex) may be discredited, but new myths, equally dysfunctional, have evolved (e.g., Women are now too sexually aggressive; Sex should be a frivolous, recreational event; Romantic love has been replaced by technique).

A wide variety of cultural patterns, belief systems, myths, and stereotypes reinforces the sexual differences between men and women. However, the growing understanding of physiological differences [17, 18] suggests that men and women have a lot in common beyond the constraints of rigid sexual roles. Even though there are hormonal differences, different roles in procreation, and possibly different sexual cycles for men and women, it is the interaction of the physiological variables with the sociocultural and psychological developmental factors that contributes to one's sexuality and how one's sexuality need is manifested. In summary, the sexuality need cannot be generalized from the anatomical differences between men and women to the social differences and differences in personality. Likewise, the way one's sexuality need is fulfilled cannot be generalized from a person of one sex to a person of another sex, but rather through an understanding of the social and personal contexts of the individual.

The development of one's sexual role and sex-typed behavior is only one of many ways in which a person becomes socialized and interacts with his or her environment. The learning of one's sexual role varies as a complex interaction; it cannot be understood as a simple, generalized phenomenon. Gratification of the sexuality need contributes to the wholeness of a person. Frustration of the need produces stress and loss of self-esteem, and it interferes with gratification of the other needs.

The nurse is often the person most closely in contact with others during stress, illness, and even so-called wellness. Gratification of the sexuality need is basic to a person's wholeness. The nurse must use a holistic approach in assisting with gratification of that need. If nursing is to become the science of caring, interventions related to the sexuality need must be examined, tested, and evaluated to provide high-quality health care.

Significance of the Sexuality Need for the Practice of Caring

1. The sexuality need involves a person's whole personality, and it must be assessed along with the other human needs

to help a person toward wellness. People meet the sexuality need in unique, personal ways.

2. The sexuality need is a basic human need that is biological in origin but dependent on psychological development for its complete functioning; it is further affected by religious and sociocultural factors.

3. Sexual satisfaction and fulfillment depend on a man's or woman's confidence and pleasure in his or her masculinity or femininity.

4. Sexual fulfillment is related to psychological growth and development, and it culminates in the young adult stage of life, in which one gives up one's attachments to one's parents and is able to enter into an intimate, loving relationship with another person.

5. One's sexual need and sexual behavior are interwoven with one's work, play, and life, the essence of sexuality being how one relates to other people.

6. Sexual matters and sexual behavior are evaluated and treated quite differently in different societies and different ages.

7. There are conflicting norms and myths about sex in contemporary Western culture. Most of them are extreme and incompatible with day-to-day expressions of sexuality.

8. The two sexual codes that are considered universal are (a) the expectation and right of sexual intercourse between marital partners and (b) the prohibition against incestuous relations between parent and child.

9. Sexual behavior becomes a matter of concern for individuals or groups when it violates or is in conflict with cherished social expectations and values.

10. Sexual differences and sexual identity are the results of a complex interaction between the internal and external forces of a social milieu (the forces that affect one's physiological, sociocultural, religious, environmental, and psychological development).

11. Society's sexual myths and stereotypes affect the internal and external forces that determine sexual identity and the differences between men and women.

12. The human sexuality need cannot be generalized from anatomical differences between men and women, and

therefore sexual satisfaction is not obtained or understood in a simple, generalized fashion but rather from the gestalt of an individual.

13. The sexuality need is prominent at all stages of human growth and development. The nurse is often the key person in providing support, information, and assistance with sexual struggles, conflicting feelings, problems of growth and development, problems of intimacy, birth control, pregnancy, marriage, and parenthood, and alterations due to sexual identity, health-illness changes, age, and so on.

14. The science of caring requires further study and research to contribute to the knowledge that is related to assistance with gratification of the sexuality need, a major carative factor.

REFERENCES

1. Bardwick, J. M. *Psychology of Women*. New York: Harper & Row, 1971.
2. Beauvoir, S. de *The Second Sex*. Translated by H. M. Parshley. New York: Knopf, 1953.
3. Beauvoir, S. de *The Coming of Age*. Translated by P. O'Brian. New York: Putnam's, 1972.
4. Boston Women's Health Book Collective. *Our Bodies, Ourselves* (2nd ed.). New York: Simon & Schuster, 1976.
5. Broverman, I. K., Vogel, S., Broverman, D., et al. Sex role stereotypes: A current appraisal. *Journal of Social Issues* 28:59, 1972.
6. Christopherson, V., Coulter, P. P., and Wolanin, M. O. *Rehabilitation Nursing*. New York: McGraw-Hill, 1974.
7. Concept Media. *The Nature of Sleep*. Program V. Costa Mesa, California. Concept Media, 1971.
8. Ellis, A., and Abanbanel, A. *The Encyclopedia of Sexual Behavior*. New York: Hawthorn, 1961.
9. Erikson, E. H. *Childhood and Society* (2nd ed.). New York: Norton, 1963.
10. Erikson, E. H. *Identity, Youth and Crisis*. New York: Norton, 1968.
11. Fraiberg, S. H. *The Magic Years*. New York: Scribner's, 1959. P. 210.
12. Hoffman, L. W. Early childhood experiences and women's achievement motives. *Journal of Social Issues* 28:129, 1972.
13. Horner, M. Toward an understanding of achievement related conflicts in women. *Journal of Social Issues* 28:157, 1972.
14. Kimmel, D. C. *Adulthood and Aging*. New York: Wiley, 1974.

15. Kleeman, D. Activity-Inactivity Need Script. (Unpublished manuscript.) Denver: The University of Colorado School of Nursing, 1971.
16. Maslow, A. H. *Motivation and Personality.* New York: Harper & Bros., 1954.
17. Masters, W. H., and Johnson, V. *Human Sexual Response.* Boston: Little, Brown, 1966.
18. Masters, W. H., and Johnson, V. *Human Sexual Inadequacy.* Boston: Little, Brown, 1970.
19. McLuhan, M. *Understanding Media: The Extensions of Man.* New York: McGraw-Hill, 1964.
20. Mitchell, P. H. *Concepts Basic to Nursing.* New York: McGraw-Hill, 1973.
21. Murray, R., and Zentner, J. *Nursing Concepts for Health Promotion.* Englewood Cliffs, N. J.: Prentice-Hall, 1975.
22. Pfeiffer, E., and Davis, G. C. Determinants of sexual behavior in middle and old age. *Journal of the American Geriatric Society* 20:151, 1972.
23. Rubin, I. *Sexual Life After Sixty.* New York: Basic Books, 1965.
24. Rubin, I. *Sexual Life in Later Years.* New York: Sex Information and Education Council of the United States, 1970.
25. van den Berg, J. H. *Psychology of the Sickbed.* Pittsburgh: Duquesne University Press, 1966. Pp. 23–35.
26. Walberg, H. J. Physics, femininity, and creativity. *Developmental Psychology* 1:47, 1969.
27. Yamamota, K. *The Child and His Image.* Boston: Houghton Mifflin, 1972. P. 7.
28. Yeaworth, R. C., and Friedman, J. S. Sexuality in later life. *Nursing Clinics of North America* 10:565, 1975.

8. ASSISTANCE WITH THE GRATIFICATION OF THE HIGHER ORDER PSYCHOSOCIAL NEEDS

THE ACHIEVEMENT NEED

In the practice of caring, a person's need to achieve must be considered a basic human need. One's ability, capability, and opportunity to accomplish and achieve comprise a higher order need and lead to self-actualization. According to Maslow, if one's higher order needs are met, one is often less preoccupied with the lower order needs. For example, people who are ill may be less preoccupied with the elimination need, if they are able to feel esteemed and accomplished at a higher level.

The achievement need has been well defined by McClelland as "behavior aimed at satisfaction of an internal standard of excellence" [16]. That definition is good because it places the standard inside the achiever rather than establishing an external standard.

It follows from that definition that the nurse assisting with gratification of the achievement need must become familiar with the internal state of the patient in order to understand the patient's standard of excellence. What is excellent to the nurse may not seem excellent to the patient; thus it is important to assess the life space of the patient.

The goal of achievement is self-approval in performing tasks at a level of competence that satisfies one. Achievement is related to recognition and receiving positive reactions from other people, to having a social acknowledgment of skills as well as an internal sense of satisfaction.

The achievement need is also closely related to the concept of motivation. The sociocultural correlates of achievement have been studied more extensively than have any other motivational systems. The achievement motivation is a concept that applies to people and their attempts at and desires for

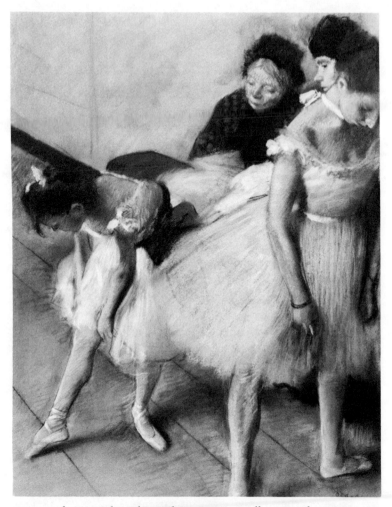

Examen de Danse, by Edgar Hilaire Degas. (Collection, The Denver Art Museum)

behavioral competence, directionality, and purposeful strivings [25].

The need for achievement is directed toward realistic accomplishments, such as when a child succeeds at play tasks (e.g., stacking blocks, drawing a tree, or building a structure).

Kagan and Moss in their Fels study [12] found that children's achievement during their early years (from birth to 2½ to 3 years of age) was not correlated with their adult behavior. However, the degree of achievement at 10 years of age was a good index to adult achievement (for both sexes).

Independent accomplishment and self-appraisal of the accomplishment are important elements in the gratification of the achievement need.

Studies have explored the origin of the achievement need [16]. The studies indicated that mothers who had a strong drive to achieve expected their sons to become independent early. For example, some mothers expected their sons to learn how to travel in the community, to make new friends, and to compete successfully with other children when they were very young.

While these studies included only mother-son relationships, it is assumed that the achievement drive can be fostered also in daughters as well as in sons. The studies show the importance of mothers' attitudes in fostering the need for achievement in their children. However, other researchers emphasize that the strength of the motivation to achieve can be changed by environmental opportunities in later childhood and by influences outside the family [26].

Achievement studies regarding sexual differences conclude that the achievement need is the same in both sexes but that men and women use different strategies to gratify the need. Men are reported to take an aggressive, active, initiating approach to achievement. Women traditionally have tried to find achievement through domestic activities, social interaction, and artistic pursuits. With the current changes in the social roles of men and women, in the future there will probably be less difference between men and women in regard to the strategies that they use to gratify the achievement need.

White wrote a classic paper on motivation that demonstrated that the theory of biological "drive" cannot explain motivation and achievement. He emphasized that motivation included such subjective and psychological variables as the novelty or complexity of a situation, its meaning for a person, interests, self-concept, esthetic qualities, play, and methods of problem solving [25].

The literature on motivation explains the achievement need

as a cognitive-affective, environmental issue, not as a physiological energy drive. There appears to be an integrative function between a person and his or her environment that motivates competency strivings and achievement (e.g., the resourcefulness of and the challenge accepted by the person, successful response to a challenge, and the desire to do well).

Strong evidence for the achievement need is shown by the activity of children in exploration and manipulation. Even children's play seems to involve finding out what can be done with the environment. Though achievement striving takes many forms, its central significance is described as the urge to attain competence in dealing with the environment [25].

As one outgrows childhood and dependency, adult standards of self-sufficiency, competence, and achievement evolve. U.S. culture has a high regard for independence, especially for men. Recent social changes and the women's movement have created more awareness of interdependence and cooperation. It appears that competency strivings and the achievement need are influenced by parental attitudes in childhood, one's subjective senses of accomplishment and environmental control, and one's resultant confidence and self-esteem. The achievement need is further enhanced by experiences that help validate the idea that certain self-sufficient behavior can be anticipated and expected through certain experiences.

According to social-learning theory [21], the achievement need can be generalized to be a function of the *expectation* (of a person about a given behavior in a given situation) that certain behavior(s) at (a) given time(s) will bring him or her the *reinforcement of values* that is needed for an internal sense of satisfaction. Other factors are the *relevance* of the event to the person and the following structures:

1. *The Opportunity Structure.* The set of values and access to opportunities desired.
2. *The Normative Structure.* The social norms about behavior. The lack of a normative structure is referred to as anomic or the state of anomie (no norms).
3. *The Social Control Structure.* Access to organized units of society that sanction behavior, such as the family, church, and school.

In regard to the framework just discussed, behavior related to the achievement need can be expressed according to Rotter's social-learning theory:

BP = f(E + RV)
(*B*ehavior *P*otential is a function of *E*xpectation plus *R*einforcement *V*alue)

A person expects that certain achievement behavior will bring the reinforcement value to satisfy an internal standard.

The formula can be applied to understanding and assessing the achievement need and assisting with its gratification for persons who are well or ill. The self-approval one seeks for performing tasks at a certain level of competence may change drastically for a person who is ill or has an altered state of functioning. A man who has farmed all his life and done heavy labor may be unable to perform those tasks with competence or satisfaction after he has had a heart attack, major surgery, or a debilitating illness or has lost a limb, a bodily structure, or a bodily function. Such a person may continue to value his former work and role but be unable to gain self-approval because he cannot achieve his former level of competence, the level that satisfies him. He might feel frustration, anger, and low self-esteem.

The practice of caring often must help people to (1) gain a more realistic view of themselves and their limitations and (2) identify tasks that they can perform at a level of competence that they find satisfying. Thus the opportunity structure as well as the normative structure may have to be reexamined. The opportunity that gives access to the values one expects may no longer be available. Likewise, the social norms about achievement may still be present in the person's social environment, but the normative structure and the shared norms of significant others might have to change (perhaps the health professional might help to create another normative structure).

Achievement is influenced by the individual's expectations of success or failure in given situations with certain behavior. If behavior that was previously successful and fulfilling to a person now results in failure, the total life space of the

experiencing person undergoes confusion. Ultimately, it
would need to be altered to prevent a situation that could
result in failure, low self-esteem, depression, helplessness, or
hopelessness.

Achievement in American society is a highly emphasized
norm. In McClelland's view [16], national and economic
growth depends in large part on the need for achievement.
Others have correlated achievement imagery in children's textbooks with the number of patents issued by the U.S. government [6].

During the nineteenth century, there was a high achievement motivation that was reinforced by the Protestant ethic
of hard work and no play. In the twentieth century the social
ethic of the United States has been described as having changed
from one of hard work and no play to one of all play [11, 12].
That assessment was supported by a decline in the number of
patents issued after 1890 [6].

The U.S. sociocultural system and its underlying patterns
affect life-styles and directly or indirectly affect the achievement need, the opportunity structure, the normative structure,
and the social control structure. Major sociocultural variables,
such as class, achievement-value differences, and sexual differences, have been reported to be associated with the achievement need.

The value differences in achievement motivation can also
be related to class differences. There is an association between
middle class values and the expectations of the middle class
for the success and future rewards that result from present
sacrifices and hard work. Lower class children may experience
less success in achievement than middle class children. That
experience would, in turn, affect the expectation that certain
behaviors would bring certain results. Lower class children
would expect little success.

The expectation of failure is a significant index to achievement. For example, the self-fulfilling prophecy of failure leads
to repeated task failure. When expectations of failure increase,
the tendency to avoid the situation that presents an opportunity for failure also increases. It is also reported that an
identification with an incompetent parent and negative

communication with a significant other can lead to a negative self-evaluation.

The literature on social class and achievement shows that middle class and upper class children score higher than lower class children on achievement motivation. That is true whether achievement is measured by performance (a measurement of actual behavior, such as persistence with challenging tests) or by a fantasy theme (e.g., by projective tests, interviewing themes, or fantasies) [16]. The finding may be related to the opportunity structure that Rotter conceptualized, or it may also be related to the normative structure and the behaviors that actually lead to an internal sense of success [16].

Margaret Mead suggested that the "conditional love" and love withdrawal patterns used in U.S. society for discipline lead to an internal sense of guilt [17]. The guilt then motivates achievement.

Different countries and different ethnic groups have different achievement values. The measure for achievement success in American society is money, whereas other countries and groups have different achievement values. The Greeks and Italians historically have valued achievement as a state of civilization of artistic and cultural accomplishments (e.g., in art, music, sculpture, and design). The Sioux Indians provide another example of a different achievement value. Among them heavy emphasis is placed on the achievement of the role of warrior and hunter.

The nurse should know about the different expectations and behaviors that are related to meeting the achievement need. They tend to vary according to sociocultural differences, value differences, and sexual differences.

The achievement need seems to be more psychologically and socioculturally determined than biologically determined. However, the various options for achievement are also related to talent and genetic endowment. The channel through which one's behaviors and accomplishments become actualized tends to be environmentally determined. The important points are that the need leads to an internal sense of satisfaction and accomplishment and it is related to social approval from others. It could be conceived as closely related to self-worth and self-concept. It is a higher order need that serves to satisfy a person's internal and external senses of competence and environmental control.

Summary
The achievement need helps one's development and growth toward self-actualization.

The assessment of achievement as a need and as a behavioral expression must be examined according to the individual's internal standard of excellence and satisfaction. The standard operates from within the person and not from outside or within another person (e.g., the health professional). However, the internal standard is closely related to a desire for social recognition.

Even though the achievement behaviors may be partially determined by genetic endowment, the strength of the motivation can be changed by environmental forces.

Achievement behavior can be conceptualized according to the social learning theory as a function of the expectation that a person places on certain behavior in a given situation that brings reinforcement value (e.g., the satisfaction of an internal sense of competence). That formulation is further determined by the person's opportunity structure, normative structure, and social control structure.

Major sociocultural variables, such as class, value differences, and sexual differences, are associated with the achievement need and its expression.

Significance of the Achievement Need for the Practice of Caring

1. In order to assess, intervene, and evaluate her or his professional assistance with gratification of the achievement need, the nurse needs to understand the dynamics and forces operating behind the need and its different forms of expression.
2. The nurse must know what variables are related to the achievement need and separate her or his own need and achievement values from the patient's need and values.

3. It is important to assess and determine the patient's achievement values from the internal frame of reference of the experiencing person.
4. The practice of caring includes problem solving to help the patient to choose alternative ways to meet his or her achievement need. That may be related to changes in the opportunity, normative, and social control structures of the patient that are dependent on the health-illness processes.
5. The nurse should never underestimate the patient's potential for achievement, even when previous methods and capabilities are no longer available.
6. The nurse must make sure that achievement expectations and pressures are derived from the patient and not from the nurse. The assessment of the nurse's achievement need and values surrounding achievement is the beginning step in separating the nurse from the patient and freeing the nurse to meet the patient at his or her own level within his or her own value system and normative and social control structures.
7. One's need for achievement is an important part of one's personal system; its growth cannot be isolated from the whole person, but it must be considered a vital part of one's development.
8. The achievement need is a higher order need that becomes more developed and controlled by one's intrapersonal and psychosocial mechanisms. As such, it is often abstract and intangible for the nurse; however, it is as important for growth, health and well-being as is any lower level, more biologically controlled, need.

THE AFFILIATION NEED

The deepest need of man is need to overcome his separateness and leave the prison of his aloneness [9].

Of all the basic needs and behavioral systems identified with living, the affiliation need comes closest to revealing the core of humanism.

A basic assumption of the affiliation need is that people need people — for help and companionship. Affiliation behavior is a universal need and the basis for humanism.

Each person, because he or she lives in society, must estab-'lish relationships with the other people in his or her environment. Every human being has the need to be accepted as a member of a human group; that need is closely related to establishing and maintaining one's identity.

The function of the affiliation need and affiliation behavior is *belonging*. To a certain degree, each person is trying to belong to a human group while also trying to maintain a certain amount of privacy. One's individuality comes from the way a person conducts his or her life in relation to other people. A broad consideration of the affiliation need is a way to examine and appreciate cooperative undertakings. Affiliation is centered on sharing, balancing privacy with intimacy, and balancing dependence-independence with interdependence.

Development and Origin of the Affiliation Need
According to theorists, clinicians, and researchers (Harlow, Prugh, Bowlby, Spitz, Erikson, Freud, Brazleton), the critical years for the establishment of the affiliation system are from birth to three years of age. Maternal and infant studies have supported that as the critical time. The system becomes more developed between the ages of two and four years of age, and it progresses to its peak during middle age. According to Cummings, the affiliation system shows a progressive decline after one retires from one's job. The decline may or may not be inherent, depending on a number of other variables, including one's previous affiliation patterns, environment, finances, age, health, interests, and abilities.

The origins and foundations of the affiliation system could be identified as (1) the union that occurs at conception, (2) the influence and environmental factors associated with birth and separation (the bonding that was allowed or not allowed to occur), (3) the selective attachment of infancy and childhood, (4) the learning and play situations provided by the parents, (5) the social, physical, and emotional interactions with parents and peers, (6) later school-age, adolescent, young-adult and middle-adult extensions of oneself with others, and (7) the resolutions of identity, intimacy, and generativity.

Dissolution or alteration of the affiliation system becomes attenuated throughout life by various forces; for example, the physical, social, health, stress, illness, and life-change forces. Later in life, the intensity and frequency of affiliation behavior may diminish. Cummings and Henry [5] point out the similarity of the social behavior of the very young and the very old.

The affiliation system develops in response to environmental stimuli; and one learns about oneself and others from the input from one's physical, social, behavioral, and emotional day-to-day environment.

The affiliation system allows feedback from others that helps to shape one's thoughts and support feelings, and to identify and reduce anxiety. If one is deprived of this input, he or she either fails to develop his or her potential or becomes detached from reality.

Gratification of the affiliation need provides the capacity for identification and role taking that helps one to be of use in one's world. Identification and role taking are the primary mechanisms by which the goal of affiliation is achieved. Identification and role taking depend on accurate, selective projection of one's own needs and feelings to external objects. The effectiveness of the process relies on the initial and consistent bonding, nurturing, and attachment behaviors between the mother and the child from infancy on.

Three basic interpersonal needs have been identified [22]. They are closely connected to the affiliation need. Those interpersonal needs are an inherent part of the affiliation system, and they form a basis for exploring interpersonal relationships. They can also serve as a focal point for nursing as the science of caring that promotes the achievement of potential within and between people.

The three interpersonal needs are [22]:

1. Inclusion. The need for identity, attention, and association with others and the need to belong; the struggle about whether one is "in" or "out," alone or together, private or

public. That need is closely related to Adler's original concepts of introversion versus extroversion [1].

2. Control. The need for autonomy; the power to influence authority. Control also refers to decision-making processes between people. The conflict is between controlling others and being controlled by others. The main concern is dominance — whether one is on the top or on the bottom and whether one is dependent or independent.

3. Affection. The need for intimate, emotional relationships between people. That interpersonal need is related to Erikson's intimacy versus isolation crisis [8], and it connotes concern with whether one is close to or distant from another human being. Affection especially includes feelings of love, tenderness, acceptance, trust, and warmth toward and from another person. It also includes other strong feelings; such as hate, anger, and sadness, in various degrees at different times.

Affiliation need behaviors are generally manifested in the way a person usually responds to being with and relating to other people in the interpersonal realm according to the three interpersonal needs. The affiliation need can be viewed as a continuum from self-concern to oneself with others. Each person has a point on a continuum where he or she feels most comfortable in relation to others. Everyone usually attempts to be included in a group, to exert some control over others, and to receive affection from others while also trying to maintain a certain amount of privacy, independence, and distance from others (see figure).

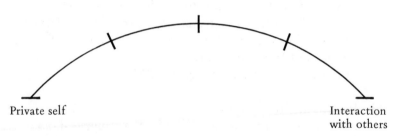

Private self   Interaction
                                                with others

The affiliation continuum.

Underlying the affiliation need and related interpersonal behavior is the assumption that people must establish relationships with other people. However, each person has a different intensity in needing others, and different mechanisms for handling interpersonal relationships. Affiliation behaviors include being accepted, understood, recognized, and liked for one's self. The motivation for the affiliation system is the avoidance of the feeling of being alone, being "cut off" or alienated from others. Belonging and relating to another person extends one's existence beyond the boundaries of the self.

The affiliation need is a part of one's cooperative undertakings and patterned interactions with the other members of a group. However, affiliation behavior may vary, depending on the kinds of social group experiences.

There are two kinds of social groups: (1) primary groups and (2) secondary groups. A primary social group provides humans with emotional security and social controls, and in most instances it refers to the nuclear family group. A nuclear family is usually composed of a mother, father, son, and(or) daughter, but that composition is changing, and a primary social group may be defined differently, depending on one's culture, life-style, current trends, social movements, and so on. For example, there are the nuclear family groups (mother, father, children) and the extended family groups (immediate family plus grandparents, in-laws, or other relatives). Both the nuclear and the extended families are primary social groups. Other people who are not related but who live as a family (such as in a commune) also belong to a primary group. Within the primary group, regardless of its members, "home" is an important symbol of stability and security. Within the primary group, the roles of its members are traditionally defined and accepted according to the current cultural and social trends of the society or country. The categories of behavior that make up affiliation patterns in a primary group are: (1) living with another (others), (2) cooperating with another (others), (3) establishing a healthy emotional and physical environment, (4) establishing a parent-child bond, and (5) nurturing and accepting others (especially children).

The significance of the primary family group for early establishment of the social affiliation system is pointed out by
Bowlby:

Actual physical separation from the mother in early childhood, to the
extent that it involves absence or loss of a relationship of dependency
with a mother figure, will have an adverse effect on personality development, particularly with respect to capacity for forming and maintaining
satisfactory object relations [4].

The secondary group provides humans with opportunities
for relationships outside the confines of the primary family
group. Affiliation relationships are established in the community with extra-familial groups (e.g., church, school, peers,
colleagues, neighbors, and business, social and recreational
contacts).

The categories of behaviors that make up the affiliative
behaviors of secondary group relationships include (1) forming friendships and (2) sharing, associating, working, and join-
ing with others. Those affiliative behaviors can lead to
humanitarian services through community, civic, professional,
religious, or charitable organizations. They allow one to
extend oneself beyond one's immediate self. They are related
to altruism and Erikson's maturity development of generativity, or providing for another generation.

Sharing in primary and secondary group relationships is a
focus of affiliation, and it serves as nourishment that enables
humans to develop and maintain contact with reality.

In research, films, and autobiographies, three things happen
to a person who is isolated from other people [24]:

1. The "pain" of the isolation experience. Prisoners of war
   have reported that they preferred torture to isolation from
   other people.
2. A strong tendency to dream, think, and, occasionally, hallu-
   cinate about other people.
3. If the person who is isolated is not occupied or distracted,
   he or she usually enters a state of withdrawal, suffering,
   apathy, diminished growth and development, and even
   failure to thrive [2, 4, 23, 24, 29].

Various models are used to explain patterns of behavior that express the affiliation need.

1. According to Reisman's *"Lonely Crowd" model* [19], there are three social character types: (a) the tradition-directed type, (b) the inner-directed type, and (c) the other-directed type.
2. The *Adlerian model* [1] is based on social extroversion-introversion determination as measured by the Minnesota Multiphasic Personality Inventory. The term socially extroverted describes a high-affiliation or people-dependent person. The term socially introverted describes a low-affiliation person, one who is more dependent on social surrogates, such as books, TV, theater, movies, animals, and so on. A "mixed" scorer, according to Adler, is non-dominant in either extroversion or introversion; he or she is in-between and uses both behaviors with relative uniform frequency.
3. *Cumming's social life sphere model* [5] is another model that helps to explain different expressions of the affiliation need. In that model, the individual affiliation patterns are captured by one's social life space and the frequency of one's participation in that life space. That fact is particularly relevant to understanding the elderly person's affiliation expression. Using Cumming's model, one must assess the person's social life space *and* the person's frequency of participation to be accurate. It may also be appropriate to understand how either the person's social life space *or* the person's frequency of participation has changed.

The affiliation need and affiliation behaviors are affected by health-illness. When a person is worried about his or her health or is actually ill, often he or she has decreased contact with others, including his or her family (the primary support system for the affiliation need), as well as significant others. Decreased feelings of belonging can result from such withdrawal or disengagement, even though it may be a necessary coping mechanism for the person.

The altered affiliation behaviors can in turn lead to loss of contact with day-to-day events, resulting in some degree of isolation, deprivation, and disruption of patterned behaviors and routine activities. The excerpt from van den Berg's book (pp. 151—155) that is related to the activity-inactivity need is relevant to understanding how the affiliation need is affected by even minor health problems.

Additional illness that may cause any structural or functional impairment of the body causes physical and mental discomfort that increases one's focus on oneself. Whenever one has an increased focus on oneself, one is less able to focus on the concerns or needs of others or to move beyond oneself in one's coping or growth. In that sense, the lower order needs become primary to the person, and they inhibit or preclude gratification of higher level needs. The person may be deprived of meaningful relationships with other people, which is vital to the maintenance of one's well-being and humanness.

Regardless of the life situation that provides input to a person (e.g., worry, illness, loss, change, or fear), when the person's capacity to focus on others is reduced, his or her usual affiliation behaviors change and he or she suffers frustration that is related to gratification of the affiliation need. When there is a *quantitative decrease* — and one wants fewer than the usual number of people around — one's social space and social sphere contract. At the same time, there is a corresponding *qualitative increase* regarding the value of the people around. Fewer people who are special and meaningful to a person are more satisfying to a person than many people who have only a superficial relationship to the person. Although ordinarily a person's affiliation need may be balanced, health-illness coping processes and the treatment regimens may drastically affect quantitative and qualitative concerns of the person.

A hospitalized person may be denied the few qualitative relationships that he or she desires and instead have an increase in limited superficial relationships with a variety of health care workers. "They have swabbed me clear of my loving associations" [18]. The result is the opposite of what is required for gratification of the affiliation need during health-illness changes. Just when a person has a reduced capacity for the company of others, he or she has a heightened need for the company of others. The others often include nurses, and therefore, the quality of the interaction with the nurse during illness is vital to gratification of the affiliation need. Such awareness and understanding of the affiliation need is necessary to guide and direct nursing care. Knowledge of the affiliation need contributes to high-quality holistic care that gratifies both lower order and higher order needs.

Significance of the Affiliation Need for the
Practice of Caring

1. The affiliation need is a universal human need, and it forms the core of humanism.
2. The affiliation need is the basis for one's cooperative undertakings and the foundation for relating to oneself and others.
3. Different models help to explain different expressions of the affiliation need. However, affiliation behaviors are manifested differently by different people on a continuum of the need for privacy-separateness with oneself to the need for intimacy-closeness with others. That is balanced by cooperative undertakings with other people for interdependence and sharing.
4. The origin and development of affiliation behavior is dependent on the early (infancy) experience of a warm, intimate, and continuous relationship with a mother figure.
5. The primary group family structure best provides the relationship and environment that are necessary for development and maintenance of the affiliation need.
6. The three basic interpersonal needs (inclusion, control, and affection) are inherent parts of the development of the affiliation need and the affiliation behaviors.
7. The affiliation need and the affiliation behaviors are affected by health-illness changes and by treatment regimens.
8. During health-illness changes, a person has a reduced capacity for others, with a heightened need for high-quality interaction with others.

9. That combined interaction (the reduced capacity for others and the heightened need for others) has profound implications for the practice of caring and the carative factors the nurse brings to bear in assistance with gratification of the affiliation need.

REFERENCES

1. Adler, A. *The Practice and Theory of Individual Psychology.* New York: Harcourt, 1927.
2. Bowlby, J. Grief and mourning in infancy and early childhood. *Psychoanalytic Study of the Child* 15:52, 1960.
3. Bowlby, J. *Child Care and the Growth of Love.* Baltimore: Penguin, 1963.
4. Bowlby, J. *Attachment.* Attachment and Loss, vol. I. New York: Basic Books, 1969.
5. Cummings, E., and Henry, W. E. *Growing Old: The Process of Disengagement.* New York: Basic Books, 1961.
6. DeCharms, R., and Moeller, G. H. Values expressed in children's readers: 1800-1950. *Journal of Abnormal and Social Psychology* 64:136, 1962.
7. Engel, G. L. *Psychological Development in Health and Disease.* Philadelphia: Saunders, 1962.
8. Erikson, E. H. *Childhood and Society.* New York: Norton, 1950.
9. Fromm, E. *Escape from Freedom.* New York: Rinehart, 1941.
10. Fromm, E. *Man for Himself.* New York: Rinehart, 1947.
11. Harlow, H. F., and Zimmerman, R. R. Affectional responses in the infant monkey. *Science* 130:431, 1959.
12. Kagan, J., and Moss, H. A. *Birth to Maturity: A Study in Psychological Development.* New York: Wiley, 1962.
13. Mahler, M. S., Pine, F., and Bergman, A. *The Psychological Birth of the Human Infant.* New York: Basic Books, 1975.
14. Maslow, A. H. *Motivation and Personality* (2nd ed.). New York: Harper & Row, 1970.
15. McClelland, D. C. Testing for competence rather than "intelligence." *American Psychologist* 28:1, 1973.
16. McClelland, D. C., Atkinson, J. W., Clark, R. A., and Lowell, E. A. *The Achievement Motive.* New York: Appleton-Century-Crofts, 1953.
17. Mead, M. *Sex and Temperament in Three Primitive Societies.* New York: Morrow, 1953.
18. "Tulips" in *Ariel* by Sylvia Plath. Copyright © 1962 by Ted Hughes. By permission of Harper & Row, Publishers, Inc.

19. Reisman, D. *The Lonely Crowd: A Study of the Changing American Character.* New Haven, Conn.: Yale University Press, 1950.
20. Rotter, J. B. *Social Learnings and Clinical Psychology.* Englewood Cliffs, N.J.: Prentice-Hall, 1954.
21. Rotter, J. B. Some implications of a social learning theory, for prediction of goal directed behavior from testing procedures. *Psychological Review* 67:301, 1960.
22. Schutz, W. C. *Joy Expanding Human Awareness.* New York: Grove, 1967.
23. Spitz, R. Anaclitic depression. *Psychoanalytic Study of the Child* 1:53, 1945.
24. Spitz, R. A. The role of ecological factors in emotional development in infancy. *Child Development* 21:145, 1949.
25. White, R. W. Motivation reconsidered: The concept of competence. *Psychological Review* 66:297, 1959.
26. White, R. W. *The Enterprise of Living* (2nd ed.). New York: Holt, Rinehart and Winston, 1976.
27. Wolfenstein, M. The emergence of fun morality. *Journal of Social Issues* 7:15, 1951.
28. Wolfenstein, M. Trends in infant care. *American Journal of Orthopsychiatry* 23:120, 1953.
29. Zubek, J. P. (ed.). *Sensory Deprivation: Fifteen Years of Research.* New York: Appleton-Century-Crofts, 1969.

9. ASSISTANCE WITH THE GRATIFICATION OF THE HIGHER ORDER INTRAPERSONAL-INTERPERSONAL NEED

THE SELF-ACTUALIZATION NEED

> *... every person is in certain respects:*
> a. *like all other persons (universal norms)*
> b. *like some other persons (group norms)*
> c. *like no other persons (idiosyncratic norms)* [9]

According to Allport [2], Maslow [10, 11, 12], Rogers [13] and others, every person has some internal striving to become, to grow, and to fulfill himself or herself. That striving is referred to as the need for self-actualization. In certain theories of psychology, it is thought to be a universal higher order need. At the same time, the need is manifested in unique, distinct ways by different people. In this book it is labeled as the highest order need. It is related to the internal striving expressed by Siddhartha [8]:

> ... what was it they could not teach you? And he thought: It was the Self, the character and nature of which I wished to learn .... Truly nothing in the world has occupied my thoughts as much as the Self ... that I am one and am separated and different from everybody else, that I am Siddhartha ....

It is the internal need that each person has to mature to the highest level of himself or herself. It is thought to be dependent on gratification of the lower order needs, on environmental and interpersonal factors, and on the unique intrapersonal characteristics of each person.

Before self-actualization can be understood as a human need, it must be realized that it is closely related to the values and *meanings perceived as relevant and important to oneself* [2]. Values inherent to seeking self-actualization are "matters

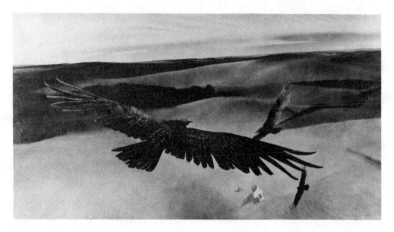

Soaring, by Andrew Wyeth. (Collection, Shelburne Museum, Shelburne, Vermont)

of internal importance" to a person rather than facts [16]. It is a person's desire for self-fulfillment, to become everything he or she is capable of becoming. The higher order needs (achievement, extended affiliation, and self-actualization) emerge only when the lower order needs have been gratified. However, when a person's lower and higher order needs are gratified, a greater value is usually placed on the higher order needs [10, 12].

In Maslow's original work on self-actualization, carefully selected persons were studied, and an extremely high standard for evaluating self-actualization was used [10, 12]. But for the purposes of this book — identifying self-actualization as a need that the nurse assists in gratifying — it is perhaps more appropriate to think of self-actualization as a "composite dimension of growth along which people move, with wide individual differences in how far they go" [15].

It is important to emphasize that in nursing care, gratification of the lower order needs produces more objective, tangible results for both the nurse and the patient, whereas "higher need gratification produces more desirable subjective results, i.e., more profound happiness, serenity, and richness of the inner life" [10]. From that perspective, the pursuit and gratification of the higher order needs represent a general trend

toward health — as Maslow says, a trend away from psychopathology. Gratification of the lower order needs alone cannot produce the high-level wellness and health that are associated with self-actualization. Feelings of relief and relaxation
may result from gratification of the lower order needs, but
not the satisfaction that is associated with one's highest level
of maturity, growth, and self-fulfillment.

Seeking self-actualization represents a movement toward
health because the more self-actualized a person is, the higher
is his or her quality of living. The works of Maslow, Rogers,
and Allport [2, 10, 11, 13] allow for that postulate. A high
quality of living is associated with a high degree of self-awareness, internal motivation, and an internal locus of control. It
provides one with the ability to face life directly, with its pain,
joys, and sorrows.

Health is related to a large degree to the quality of living,
and it is dependent on self-awareness and self-acceptance. A
goal in nursing often is helping others to reach higher levels
of self-actualization, whether doing so requires further understanding and acceptance of a disease and its consequences or
further understanding of the patient's life stresses and living
patterns and how they contribute to health maintenance and
the onset of disease.

Perhaps it is idealistic and unrealistic for persons to work
toward self-actualization as the highest level of gratification
of needs, but it is a worthwhile goal for health care. It is a
real human need, the gratification of which nursing should
consider as a carative factor. Assistance with gratification of
the self-actualization need often requires changes in the external environment to make it possible. At the same time, the
pursuit and gratification of the need are active concerns in
contemporary society, which places a greater emphasis on
individualism, self-awareness, and self-growth.

The self-actualization need is related to Erikson's concept
of generativity, which applies to the mature adult. Even
though there is an inherent conflict between one's *intra*personal
development (self-actualization) and one's *inter*personal (societal) development (or generativity), the two are intricately
connected. Maslow identified self-actualized persons as those

who "strongly focused on problems outside themselves" and
who had "some mission in life, some task to fulfill." Erikson
proposed that the truly mature person was concerned with
establishing and guiding the next generation. The following
paragraph summarizes Erikson's attitude:

Man's capacity for imagination, reason, and conscience make it possible
and necessary for him to elevate this generativity to higher cultural,
ethical and religious levels. Generativity is not only the instinctive
source behind biological procreation and care, it is also the ground for
man's higher attempts to create a total environment ecologically supportive of the general health . . . of the entire human species [6].

In spite of an inclination to view self-actualization and generativity as being at variance with each other, the two factors
are inherently related to high-level wellness and health. In
that sense it is acknowledged that no person can be fully self-
actualized without some degree of dedication to other people.

SELF-ACTUALIZATION CHARACTERISTICS
In categorizing the human needs, the distinction between the
lower order needs and the higher order needs was made with
the intent to acknowledge self-actualization as the ultimate
human need. I consider the highest level of health to be a
subjective state of awareness — recognition of one's own
needs, behavior, desires, and motivations, and achievement of
control over one's actions. The higher order achievement and
affiliation needs are much closer to self-actualization than are
the lower order needs. To promote the highest level of health,
the practice of nursing must be attentive to both lower order
and higher order needs.

Self-actualization, as Maslow conceptualized it, consists of
different qualities that can be attributed to self-actualizing
people. The qualities are *cognitive qualities, interpersonal
qualities,* and *spontaneity* and *autonomy* [15].

Within the cognitive classification, self-actualizing people
have a "more efficient perception of reality and more comfortable relations with it." Such people's perceptions are more
accurate, and they are not distorted by desires, anxiety, or

rigidity. Self-actualizing people are "problem-centered rather than ego-centered." They are capable of rising above small things, and they "impart a certain serenity and lack of worry over immediate concerns that makes life easier, not only for themselves but for all who are associated with them." The carative factor interpersonal teaching-learning can assist with the cognitive part of self-actualization.

Spontaneity refers to behavior that is simple, natural, and genuine. Self-actualizing people are described as spontaneous in both their behavior and their inner thoughts. Self-actualization is described as a continued "freshness of appreciation," with a capacity to enjoy good and beautiful things. Even mystical feelings have value and meaning. Spontaneity can be encouraged by the nurse who is open and who encourages others to be open.

The interpersonal characteristics of self-actualizing persons have already been related to Erikson's concept of generativity. White related them to the kind of social interest that Adler identified — as sympathy and involvement with other people and a genuine desire to help them [15]. Self-actualizing people are intimate with a small number of people and therefore have no time for many deep relationships. Self-actualizing people are believed to be high in acceptance of themselves and others in spite of limitations and imperfections. That acceptance can be encouraged by using the first carative factors instillation of a humanistic-altruistic value system and the development of a helping-trust relationship. Those in turn promote acceptance of others.

The people Maslow studied cared little for trivial social interactions, and they often enjoyed privacy. That interpersonal realm of self-actualization is closely related to the affiliation need and affiliation behavior. Just as an ill person seems to require quality and depth in his or her relationships, with only a few interpersonal contacts, the self-actualizing person may be closer to the privacy end of the affiliation continuum provided that the interactions that he or she chooses are genuine.

The other quality associated with Maslow's concept of self-actualization is *autonomy*. White [15] gave that quality two specific headings: (1) autonomy, independence of culture and environment and (2) autonomy, resistance to enculturation. In Maslow's view, self-actualizing people depend less on external sources of satisfaction and more on "their own potentialities and latent resources." That trait provides an internal sense of control and acceptance of life, with its frustrations and pain. The concept is further developed by Maslow, who emphasizes that such persons "resist enculturation and maintain a certain inner detachment from the culture in which they are immersed." It is somewhat akin to the concept of freedom developed by John Dewey and Abraham Heschel; that is, to be free, one must be disciplined and attain a degree of independence [5, 7].

Self-actualization includes an inner freedom and control over one's life to the extent that people are ruled by the laws of their own characters rather than by the rules of society. Of course, the degree of detachment a person can have from society and still be productive and constructive is a delicate matter. Dewey indicated that a person's power to grow depended on his or her need for others [4].

Self-actualization is a form of personality growth. Although it is subjective and intrapersonal, it depends on one's concern and need for others.

Self-actualization does not mean only emancipation from society's demands; it includes the balance between oneself and society that the self-actualizing person attains. It does not mean self-immersion, nor does it mean that a person is controlled by external forces.

Perhaps the greater danger to one's humanness in modern society is the loss of one's self and the loss of one's capacity and freedom to be oneself. New forces that have emerged to regulate actions range from the subliminal techniques of advertising to the big government and mass media campaigns that tell people how to use their time.

GROWTH ENCOURAGEMENT

In the practice of nursing as the science of caring, assistance with the self-actualization need is an important carative factor.

If the nurse has a human need perspective in her or his caring, both lower order and higher order needs are considered. The nurse does not stop with assistance in the gratification of the lower order needs. She or he has a human and social responsibility to move beyond the patient's immediate, specific needs and help the patient to reach his or her highest level of growth, maturity, and health. Nursing's most important goal is the promotion of self-actualization.

The nurse has an obligation in regard to her or his own level of development in order to promote higher level growth in others. In that context the nurse can cultivate the ability in herself or himself and others to be aware of one's own needs and to recognize one's own inner longings for growth and development. That establishes the foundation for making free and rational decisions, it places a person in control over his or her life and its events, and it bestows the ability to accept reality without undue anxiety and misperceptions.

The concept of self-actualization requires an existential view that includes the belief that a person is capable of growth and can become more fully "human." It is a belief that people have responsibility in their own existences and are capable of continually unfolding potentialities and strength. Whether a person is self-actualized may not be as important as the belief that he or she can be self-actualized and whether he or she responds to nursing encounters that promote that idea.

The concept of self-actualization involves an individualized approach to people. Within each person is a unique and idiosyncratic character structure. Self-actualization, even if it is universal, is by definition actualization of *one* self; no two selves are alike. Even though Maslow found similarities in the people he classified as self-actualized, each person developed in a unique way.

The implications of self-actualization and high levels of wellness have not been examined. The clinical and theoretical study of the self-actualizing person, so far as it has been pursued, indicates the special status of lower order and higher order needs. The healthy life is supported and promoted by the gratification of human needs. Health is primarily the domain of nursing. Additional study, practice, and research are required for nursing to include the gratification of higher order needs as a carative factor; but, for now, it suffices to establish the conceptual basis for human needs as a pertinent concern of nursing as the science of caring.

THE SIGNIFICANCE OF THE CARATIVE FACTOR ASSISTANCE WITH THE GRATIFICATION OF THE SELF—ACTUALIZATION NEED

1. Self-actualization is considered the highest order human need, in which one seeks development of one's potentialities and self-fulfillment.
2. Even though self-actualization is designated in this book an *intra*personal need that is uniquely manifested for each person, it is closely related to one's *inter*personal development, maturity, and generativity.
3. The lower order needs (e.g., the food and fluid, elimination, and ventilation needs) are more localized, tangible, and limited than are the higher order needs, especially the self-actualization need. Whereas gratification of the lower order needs produces more objective results for the nurse and others, gratification of the higher order needs (e.g., the achievement, affiliation, and self-actualization needs) produces more desirable subjective results, (e.g., happiness, contentment, integrity, and richness of one's inner life) [10, 11].
4. The practice of nursing as the science of caring requires that the nurse help the patient to gratify his or her needs in the order of their importance — from the lower order needs to the higher order. The nurse should help to gratify as many needs as she or he can.
5. Self-actualized people have achieved the highest levels of growth, maturity, and self-fulfillment. Self-actualization can be equated with high levels of wellness and health.
6. The practice of caring has a social and human responsibility to promote high order growth in oneself and in others.

7. The studies of self-actualized persons show that the gratification of the lower order and the higher order needs promotes health — "of the entire human species" [3]. In that sense, nursing study, practice, and research could benefit from additional work related to gratification of higher order needs, and the resultant movement toward health.

REFERENCES

1. Adler, A. *The Practice and Theory of Individual Psychology.* Harcourt, Brace, 1929.
2. Allport, G. W. *The Person in Psychology.* Boston: Beacon, 1968.
3. Browning, D. S. *Generative Man: Psychoanalytic Perspectives.* Philadelphia: Westminster, 1973. P. 146.
4. Dewey, J. *Democracy and Education.* New York: Macmillan, 1916. Pp. 41–53.
5. Dewey, J. *Human Nature and Conduct.* New York: Holt, Rinehart and Winston, 1922.
6. Erikson, E. H. *Childhood and Society* (2nd ed.). New York: Norton, 1963.
7. Herschel, A. J. *The Insecurity of Freedom.* New York: Farrar, Straus, & Giroux, 1966. Pp. 14–21.
8. Hesse, H. *Siddhartha.* Translated by Hilda Rosner. New York: New Directions, 1951.
9. Kluckhohn, C. M., Murray, H. A., and Schneider, D. M. (eds.). *Personality in Nature, Society and Culture.* New York: Knopf, 1953. P. 53.
10. Maslow, A. H. *Motivation and Personality.* New York: Harper & Bros., 1954.
11. Maslow, A. H. *Toward a Psychology of Being* (2nd ed.). Princeton, N.J.: Van Nostrand, 1968.
12. Maslow, A. H. *Motivation and Personality* (2nd ed.). New York: Harper & Row, 1970.
13. Rogers, C. R. Toward a Science of the Person. In T. W. Wann (ed.), *Behaviorism and Phenomenology.* Chicago: University of Chicago Press, 1964.
14. White, R. W. *Lives in Progress* (3rd ed.). New York: Holt, Rinehart and Winston, 1975.
15. White, R. W. *The Enterprise of Living* (2nd ed.). New York: Holt, Rinehart and Winston, 1976.
16. Whitehead, A. N. *Science and the Modern World.* New York: Macmillan, 1925.

10. ALLOWANCE FOR EXISTENTIAL-PHENOMENOLOGICAL FACTORS

The carative factor allowance for existential-phenomenological factors acknowledges the foundation of the separateness and identity of each person. The carative factor rests on the personal, subjective experience of the person as the foundation for understanding. It helps the nurse to turn inward, to the self as the source of values and strengths. In the day-to-day living that brings problems, struggles, pain, and suffering to so many people, the existential-phenomenological factors bring personal meaning to the human predicament.

Dealing with another person as he or she *is* and in relation to what he or she would *like* to be or could be is a matter of existential-phenomenological concern for the nurse who practices the science of caring. Nursing as a profession gives serious attention to the health-illness concerns of people. Nursing practice includes the concept of the wholeness of a person. It addresses itself to the "lower nature" (i.e., the lower order human needs) as well as the "higher nature" (i.e., the higher order needs, the "god-likeness"). On the whole, while nursing has addressed itself to the whole nature of people, it has often dichotomized the nature of the needs (into lower order needs and higher order needs). An existential-phenomenological perspective teaches the nurse that neither of those aspects of human nature can be repudiated; they can only be integrated, because they simultaneously define characteristics of human nature [11].

Probably no profession (unless perhaps the religious ministry) is more aware than nursing that some human problems are insoluble. The human predicament that results from various health conditions and coping with illness is often a gap between human aspirations and human limitations.

Empirically, nursing is well acquainted with the great human variable of strength (courage, determination, persistence — or

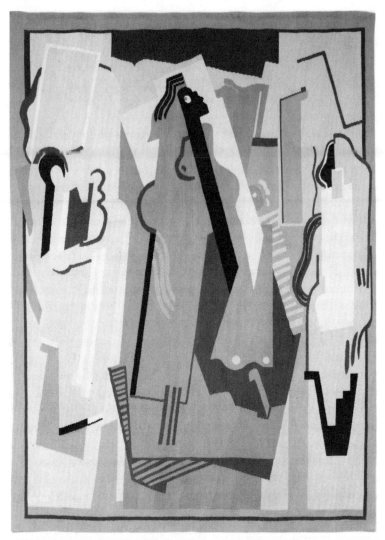

Autorité Spirituelle et Pourvoir-Aubusson, by Albert Gliezes. (Collection, The Denver Art Museum)

whatever one chooses to call it) that accounts for remarkable coping with, adjusting to, overcoming, or accepting one's health-illness condition. When a person is faced with a conflict between his or her aspiration and limitations, his or her unique responses do not fit into any categories of medical science.

It is not medical science but nursing science that can teach one that the best way to understand another human being is to get into his or her *Weltanschauung,* * to look at the world through his or her eyes [11]. In many instances, only the existential-phenomenological view can account for the mysteries of human life and people's unique ways of coping with the human predicaments. Many people know instances of tragedy's bringing profound depth and meaning to one's life rather than the shallowness and superficiality of a diminished level of living.

Such profundity of living is shown in the existential struggles of Viktor Frankl [5]. A prisoner in concentration camps for a long time, Frankl struggled to find a reason to live after his release. His entire family, except for his sister, had died in the camps. He had lost every possession, had had every value attacked, had suffered from hunger, cold, brutality, and the fear of extermination [5]. Yet he was able to find meaning and responsibility in his life.

In contrast with Frankl's involuntary suffering and the existential meaning he discovered in life is the aristocratic, luxury-filled life of Tolstoy, who subjected himself to voluntary suffering and deprivation in order to find meaning and responsibility in his life. Although Tolstoy was not considered an existentialist in his time, the beliefs he held in the early 1800s are closely related to the later existential views of Sartre, Camus, Heidegger, Husserl, Buber, and others [4, 7, 8, 12].

The concepts of existentialism and phenomenology are closely related, and they support a subjective appreciation of the inner world of the experiencing person. As nurses know, at least on some level, a patient may have human problems that may at first be "completely hidden from our eyes" [6, 9]. In order to find solutions to hidden problems it may be necessary to find meanings that may have little direct connection to the patient's experiences. In other words, the human problems that the nurse encounters may not be directly related to the patient's external human predicament, but they may be related to the patient's internal human predicament as he or she experiences the world.

*Philosophy of life, world outlook, views, creed, ideology [2].

Existential-phenomenological factors help to account for the success or failure of a sufferer (whether the origin of the suffering is external or internal) to find meaning and a sense of responsibility in his or her existence. The unseen, and sometimes unknown, psychological events that offer meaning to the human predicament are such things as love for one's children, a belief in another life, a talent to be used, or a memory worth preserving [11].

The incorporation of existential-phenomenological factors into the science of caring helps the nurse to understand (and perhaps to explain) the meaning a patient finds in life. It is a philosophical approach to viewing the human predicament rather than a technique of any sort. Using such a philosophy and awareness in a nursing situation can help the nurse personally and professionally; it can be a guiding influence in turning tragedy and other difficult life experiences into strengths.

As mentioned, existentialism and phenomenology are interrelated. The leaders of existentialism ofen played important roles in phenomenology. Köhler, Koffka, Wertheimer, and others founded Gestalt psychology and adopted phenomenology as a method of study. Heidegger and Husserl, both of whom are considered existentialists, were closely associated with modern phenomenology; Husserl, in fact, is considered its founder [6].

TERMINOLOGY
Since the terms phenomenology and existentialism — and their significance to nursing study, practice, and research — are perhaps not widely known in nursing, they are defined and discussed in the following paragraphs.

Phenomenology is a description of the data or the givens of an immediate situation that help one to understand the phenomenon in question. A phenomenological orientation to nursing has the following properties [16]:

1. It concerns itself with the unique subjective and objective experiences of the individual (or family or group).
2. It adopts a holistic, gestalt attitude toward the understanding of one's self and others.

3. It holds the individuality of the person as its most important concern.
4. It values people because they are inherently good and capable of development.
5. It values the total person context or gestalt as a more important determinant of health-illness care than the patient's bacteria, organic pathogens or disorders alone.

Phenomenology refers to an emphasis on understanding people from the way things appear to them — from their own phenomenal world. The person and his or her internal and external experience are the focuses of all experience. The totality of experience at any given moment constitutes a phenomenal field. The phenomenal field is the individual's (family's, group's) frame of reference, and it can truly be known only by the experiencing person. But the nurse seeks to understand the individual's internal reference point even though it can never be perfectly known [16].

Phenomenology, as understood in Gestalt psychology, has been used for "investigating phenomena of such psychological processes as perceiving, learning, remembering, thinking, and feeling" [6], but it has not been used in nursing studies to investigate the experiencing person's coping with health-illness. It offers a rich methodology to the science of caring.

Existential psychology has been defined as "an empirical science of human existence which employs the method of phenomenological analysis [6]. That method consists of describing or explaining experience in the language of experience. A significant aspect of the method is the deriving of data that indicate that a person "really feels understood" by another. The experience of "really feeling understood" is necessary for the nurse to establish and communicate to other people. According to a phenomenological-existential perspective, "really feeling understood" is:

"a perceptual emotion Gestalt: /A subject perceiving/that a person/ coexperiences/what things mean to the subject/and accepts him,/feels, initially, relief from existential loneliness/and gradually, safe experiential communion/with that person/and with that which the subject perceives this person to represent" [15].

PHENOMENOLOGICAL METHOD

Table 10-1 includes the results of an *intrasubjective* validation experience used in an existential case study by Van Kaam [15]. He gathered spontaneous descriptions from high school and college students of situations in which they felt they were understood by someone and of how they felt in each of the situations. He then identified the basic structure that emerged when one tried to explain the phenomenon of "being understood." After unrelated items were eliminated and other items were combined, nine items remained.

Table 10-1. Constituents of Experience of "Really Feeling Understood" and Percentages of People Expressing Constituents

Constituents of the Experience of "Really Feeling Understood"	Percentage of People Studied Expressing Constituents
Perceiving signs of understanding from the other person	87
Perceiving that the other person co-experiences what things mean to one	91
Perceiving that the other person accepts one	86
Feeling satisfaction	97
Feeling relief initially	93
Feeling relief initially from experiential loneliness	89
Feeling safe in a relationship with the understanding person	91
Feeling safe, experiential communion with the understanding person	86
Feeling safe, experiential communion with what the understanding person is perceived to represent	64

Source: Hall and Lindzey [6].

The items of "really feeling understood" are closely related to the conditions necessary for a helping relationship. These are helpful data for nursing to explore because of the therapeutic need to work with people and communicate to them that they are understood. Therefore the *intrasubjective validation* method related to existentialism and phenomenology holds much promise as a research method in nursing.

Another method of phenomenological analysis used in existential research is called *intersubjective validation.* It consists of having trained phenomenologists independently describe the same phenomenon and then compare the results. Nurse researchers may utilize that method effectively in care situations in which they are constantly observing a patient's behavior under stressful conditions. The validity of this method is determined experimentally by testing hypotheses deduced (or induced) from care situations. For example, one might predict from the general assumption that "humans always maintain some kind of dialogue with their environment" that sensory deprivation will result in imaginings, fantasies, and hallucinations. As mentioned in the discussion of the activity-inactivity need, the prediction has been confirmed by sensory deprivation studies [18].

If nursing considers the intersubjective validation method from an inductive position, the nurse could empirically observe the phenomena of fantasies and hallucinations in patients in whom sensory deprivation occurs (e.g., those in coronary care units and isolation rooms), record the presence of such phenomena, and fit them into the general assumption that they are a way of maintaining dialogue with the environment. Existential-phenomenological research in nursing may extend the method further by attempting to verify the phenomenological description of the situation for the patient and to test out intervention strategies to promote a more healthful environmental dialogue for the patient rather than a fantasized relationship with his or her environment.

REALM OF NURSING CARE
Although the concepts of existentialism and phenomenology may be undeveloped in nursing, continued attention to them and the relevant research strategies hold much promise for nursing as the science of caring. The nature of the human

being in the world is the whole of one's existence, which is made up of:

1. One's biological or physical surroundings
2. One's human environment
3. The person himself or herself, including his or her body

Nursing care encompasses all three regions of the world in which the human being has existence. In addition, nursing care is concerned with man's possibilities (or *being-beyond-the-world*, in existential terms), which include assisting others to actualize their potentialities to live an authentic life. That is related to assistance with gratification of higher order needs, specifically self-actualization. In existential terms, "In other words, man is to accept all his life-possibilities, he is to appropriate and assemble them to a free authentic own self no longer caught in the narrowed-down mentality of an anonymous, inauthentic everybody. Man's freedom consists in becoming ready for accepting and letting be all that is . . ." [3].

EXISTENTIAL CURATIVE FACTORS

The inclusion of existential factors in a clinical sense rather than a theoretical one is found in Yalom's work [17]. Yalom included "existential factors" as one of the curative factors in his therapeutic group studies. He realized later that the original curative factors he studied were incomplete, and he constructed five items to pinpoint the existential factors. They consist of the following levels of awareness that help to account for psychological cures [17]:

1. Recognizing that life is at times unfair and unjust
2. Recognizing that ultimately there is no escape from some of life's pain and from death
3. Recognizing that no matter how close I get to other people, I still face life alone
4. Facing the basic issues of my life and death, and thus living my life more honestly and being less caught up in trivialities

5. Learning that I must take ultimate responsibility for the way I live my life no matter how much guidance and support I get from others

Interestingly, Yalom respondents ranked the entire category of "existential factors" higher than some other valued factors, such as universality, altruism, and guidance. There seems to be some evidence to support the theory that existential factors play an important but generally unrecognized role in health care.

When basic views of humanity are examined in nursing, it may come as a surprise that the profession has an existential orientation without the orientation's having been overtly acknowledged.

Often it is the existential-phenomenological carative factor that helps people cope with the human predicaments. When people have the opportunity to realize certain important but painful truths about their existences, they develop internal strength and control of their lives. Just as people learn to face their *being*, so they can come to terms with their *non-being*. In so doing, day-to-day concerns are seen in a different perspective. Trivia become less of a concern.

A nurse can never eliminate the problems of separateness and aloneness that must be confronted by each person; they cannot be resolved, they can only be known. Each person has to find his or her own way to confront the problems of existence. The nurse must confront her or his own problems of existence, and she or he can encourage and support existential awareness in others.

In that sense the nurse can care for others who are ill and restore and promote health, but the nurse cannot directly create health. The nurse is responsible for human conditions under special circumstances related to health-illness. The special circumstances often require that a person be helped to cope with the human predicament. An existential-phenomenological approach to coping is often the unrecognized variable that allows the person to transcend the human predicament. Each person has to develop *personal meaning* in his or her life. When an overt disease is present, it is often the individual perception of and response to the disease that brings relief, not the escape from the disease itself, especially when the disease is progressive or permanent. In other words, health is not a matter of feeling good or bad. Health is "at-one-ment with what really is" [8]. That view is an existential-phenomenological way to confront one's life and one's *being*.

SUMMARY

Nursing as a health profession daily confronts special circumstances and people's struggles with their own *beings* and *personal meanings* of the human predicament. At the same time, death and dying are events that the nurse commonly sees and that often cause the nurse to confront her or his own state of *being* and *non-being*. When a person is able to come to terms with his or her *non-being*, life and death are more authentic, and death is less feared and more a reality of life. It is often the existential-phenomenological carative factor that brings meaning and focus into one's personal and professional life and accounts for previously unrecognized courage and perhaps miraculous happenings in the existences of others.

Consideration and attention to the existential-phenomenological carative factor for the science of caring have exciting and unlimited possibilities for nursing study, practice, and research. The phenomenon of health and the human predicament of coping with illness are perhaps not only *best* but perhaps *only* understood from an existential-phenomenological perspective.

Because existential-phenomenological issues are varied, universal, abstract, and philosophical, I recommend that the nurse read William Barrett's *Irrational Man* [1]. It is an excellent introduction to existentialism.

This factor is the last identified carative factor that is part of nursing as the science of caring. Discussion on that factor brings to a close the discussion of the major concepts that comprise nursing. No one factor can be effective alone. The student nurse and the practicing nurse must continue to integrate the factors that effect positive health care. It is hoped that those factors give some structure and order to the

continued study, practice, and research efforts of nursing to
further develop the science of caring.

REFERENCES

1. Barret, W. *Irrational Man.* New York: Doubleday, 1962.
2. Betteridge, H. T. (ed.). *The New Cassell's German Dictionary.* New York: Funk & Wagnalls, 1958.
3. Boss, M. *Psychoanalysis and Daseinsanalysis.* New York: Basic Books, 1963.
4. Buber, M. *I and Thou* (2nd ed.). New York: Scribner's, 1958.
5. Frankl, V. E. *Man's Search for Meaning.* New York: Washington Square Press, 1963.
6. Hall, C. S., and Lindzey, G. *Theories of Personality* (2nd ed.). New York: Wiley, 1970.
7. Heidegger, M. *Being and Time.* New York: Harper & Row, 1962.
8. Hora, T. Transcendence and healing. *Journal of Existential Psychiatry* 1:501, 1961.
9. Köhler, W. *Gestalt Psychology: An Introduction to New Concepts in Psychology.* New York: Liveright, 1947.
10. Lewin, K. *A Dynamic Theory of Personality.* New York: McGraw-Hill, 1935.
11. Maslow, A. H. *Toward a Psychology of Being* (2nd ed.). Princeton, N.J.: Van Nostrand, 1968.
12. Sartre, J.-P. *Being and Nothingness.* New York: Philosophical Library, 1956.
13. Tillich, P. *The Courage to Be.* Yale University Press, 1952.
14. Tolstoy, L. *The Wisdom of Tolstoy.* New York: Philosophical Library, 1968. Translated by Huntington Smith. An abridgement L. Tolstoy, *My Religion.* London: Walter Scott, 1889.
15. Van Kaam, A. *Existential Foundations of Psychology.* Pittsburgh: Duquesne University Press, 1966. Pp. 325–326.
16. Watson, J. Supporting materials for and introduction to the new undergraduate curriculum for the University of Colorado School of Nursing. Denver, Colo., 1976.
17. Yalom, I. D. *The Theory and Practice of Group Psychotherapy* (2nd ed.). New York: Basic Books, 1975.
18. Zubek, J. P. (ed.). *Sensory Deprivation.* New York: Appleton-Century-Crofts, 1969.

III. APPLICATION OF THE CARATIVE FACTORS TO SITUATIONS THAT AFFECT HEALTH-ILLNESS

Parts I and II of this book introduced nursing students and practicing nurses to my conceptual and philosophical view of nursing as the science of caring. Ten carative factors were identified as elements that comprise the whole of nursing and contribute to the practice of the science of caring. The material that was developed in Parts I and II presented nursing as responding to human beings in altered states of health-illness from a holistic intervention perspective. Both specific, concrete carative factors and humanistic-existential, abstract carative factors were discussed. Both dimensions must be integrated for the science of caring.

The 10 carative factors described are basic to nursing. They consist of those aspects of nursing that I consider intrinsic to making a difference through nursing care.

Although the carative factors may be the essence of what comprises high level nursing care, it is also helpful for the student nurse and the practicing nurse to conceptualize various day-to-day situations to which the nurse can apply the carative factors for health care intervention. Although the carative factors apply to the care of both healthy and ill people, they lend themselves best to primary health care, or what I prefer to call holistic care.

Holistic care promotes (1) humanism, (2) health, and (3) quality living. These three states are more apt to result from the science of caring that studies, practices, and researches (1) the health-illness behaviors of persons coping with (a) stress-change, (b) developmental conflict, or (c) loss and (2) the caring intervention behaviors of nurses that are most effective in promoting humanism, health, and quality living. It is my belief (one that is supported by increasing numbers of theories and by research) that these two conditions are valid concerns for illness prevention, health promotion, and a higher level of wellness.

The science of caring encompasses these holistic variables. Nursing is in a key position to promote humanism, health, and quality living through theory and knowledge development, research, and practice.

In further pursuing the practice of the science of caring, nurses can integrate the carative factors with the various intervention behaviors that encourage patients to develop responsibility and self-control in coping with stress-change, developmental conflicts, and loss. Systematic nursing interventions to help people handle stress-changes, developmental conflicts, and loss could make major contributions to primary health care and illness prevention. The result would be close to holistic care, which reduces stress and encourages the patient to be responsible for his ongoing health. If primary nursing intervention occurs around those three human conditions (stress-change, developmental conflicts, and loss), nursing health care will be relevant to the daily circumstances of living, not simply to illness symptoms or problems. Stress-changes are normal and common, but they can affect health and result in illness onset. Illness is often related to a person's response to stress-change, development, and loss. Those states occur so often that they are usually taken for granted and no effort is made to handle them better. There is sufficient evidence now for nursing to give explicit attention to those states and related responses. Part III of this book discusses those states as circumstances that require nursing intervention for holistic primary care.

Part III first discusses the concepts of health and stress to help the student nurse and the practicing nurse to understand why nursing must address itself to the states and coping patterns related to stress-change, developmental conflict, and loss in order to give primary care.

11. HEALTH AND ITS DETERMINANTS

Over a century ago Florence Nightingale established nursing's practice focus as the assessment and promotion of the health status, assets, and health potential of human beings of all ages, nationalities, races, and varieties of human circumstances. Nursing is still trying to achieve those goals.

Health is at best an illusive concept, because (for one reason) it is an individually defined phenomenon. In general, people are considered to be in good health if they can meet the daily expectations of their family, job, and social roles. Nursing has had difficulty in defining and evaluating health outcome goals because many variables affect health. Often no clear distinction is made between health and illness, because the states are relative ones. They are not distinct absolute states. Health is a process of adapting, coping, and growing that goes on from conception to death. Health-illness operate simultaneously to stabilize and balance one's life.

Everyone agrees that health is more than the absence of disease. Some people have defined it as the presence of a sense of well-being and the absence of disease, excessive conflict, and anxiety [37]. The World Health Organization has defined health as a positive state of physical, mental, and social well-being.

Recent concepts of health relate it to dimensions of self-sufficiency, self-satisfaction, and self-care, a view that suggests that a healthy person has a high-quality, balanced life, a sense of happiness, and the ability to adapt to change. But although those "quality-of-life" and "self-satisfied" outcomes might be expected to be the results of health care delivery efforts, they are not. Despite the great increase in health expenditures and in the number of health workers over the past ten years, the nation's health has not improved as much as expected [29]. The lack of improvement may be explained by the fact that the term health connotes at least the following three elements:

1. A high level of overall physical, mental, and social functioning
2. A general adaptive-maintenance level of daily functioning
3. The absence of illness (or the presence of efforts that lead to its absence)

Because of those elements, a set of health concerns and solutions suitable to one level of health may be perceived as inappropriate to another level of health. Thus the reports of the amounts of money said to be spent for health care (perhaps hundreds of billions of dollars) are misleading. Most efforts and funds given to "health" are used for the care of the ill and for hospital expenses. Likewise, although there are more than 200 types of health workers, few are concerned with health in its broadest sense.

To further confuse the issue of health, a faulty myth has been allowed to take hold — the myth that medical care is the same as health care. Only recently has it been admitted that medical care is *not* the same as health care [57]. Indeed, some people have claimed that medical care not only does not equal health care but is even a threat to health [25]. The reason for that may be related to the fact that medical care (that provided by doctors, drugs, and hospitals), although comprising most of traditional health care, "affects [only] about 10 percent of the usual indices for measuring health: whether you live at all (infant mortality), how well you live (without illness), how long you live (adult mortality)" [57].

The potent health determinants (the remaining 90 percent of the health indices) are factors over which traditional health care has little or no control — life-style, personality, psychosocial characteristics, social conditions, and physical environment [57]. But most advancements in health care are made in traditional health care, ignoring 90 percent of the factors that affect health (see figure). To compound the problem, the health-illness issues that occur most frequently and affect the greatest number of people are those linked not to specific diseases but to psychosocial pathology. For example, illegitimate births, divorce, drug abuse, crime, violent behavior, poverty, learning difficulties, and psychological problems are all maladies that reflect some unhealthiness in society.

90% of health problems	10% of health problems
No specific treatment available; these health conditions are related to:	Treatment via drugs, doctors, and hospitalization
1. Individual life-style (smoking, exercise, worry) 2. Social conditions (income, eating habits, physiological inheritance) 3. Physical environment (air and water quality)	1. Illness 2. Disease, diagnosis 3. Surgery
Health care needs	Medical care focus

Health determinants and placement of health resources.

So although money, workers, and medical care are directed at 10 percent of health care (disease treatment), the other 90 percent of health care is ignored. An additional issue is that of who should address themselves to the disease treatment that comprises the third dimension of health (or 10 percent of the problem) and who should address themselves to the health problems of the first and second health dimensions (high-level functioning; prevention) — the remaining 90 percent of the problem.

Part of the problem with health workers is caused by the generalities, ambiguities, and various dimensions of health. Traditionally, medical care has assumed — and has been expected to assume — responsibility for the total picture. Medical care and physicians are, of course, invaluable. Since the advent of the bacteriological era in medicine, great advances have been made in the prevention, diagnosis, and treatment of disease. The confusion of health with treatment of disease is compounded by the "health-illness-medicine complex" that exists in the United States. Over the years, the definition of health has become diffused, and health has been equated with "a state of complete physical, mental and social well-being" [19]. As the definition of health changed, the definition of illness changed. Any dissatisfaction, dysfunction, or psychological problem is now an illness. Many physical states that were formerly considered normal ones are treated as illnesses

today. For example, the menopause, which was considered
normal in the 1940s, is treated as an illness today. Now that
medicine and physicians are expected to deal with all aspects
of health (even a patient's social or psychological problems),
more and more of the common and expected life events are
labeled and treated as illnesses. Society now expects more of
health care, and it demands more than health care can provide.

The terms health and illness now cover so many human
states, including physical, psychological and social states, that
no single person can be considered completely healthy or completely ill. No single profession can work at maintaining all
types of health or at treating all types of illness.

The issue of health-illness needs to be re-examined and rede-
fined. Is either health or illness an objective state defined by
medicine and society, or is it a subjective state that exists in
the mind and body of the person? I prefer the latter view of
health and illness. In explanation, an individual *person* has
the most control over his or her health and illness. From a
phenomenological perspective, who is to say who is ill and
who is healthy, except the experiencing person? One person
may have an infirmity but not think of himself or herself as ill.
Another person may have the same infirmity and think of himself or herself as very ill.

The concept of health is like the concept of a disability as
opposed to a handicap. The term disability refers to an organic, physical, or overt disorder that can be labeled. However, a
disability need not handicap a person. But a person can be
handicapped in his or her functioning without having an overt
or tangible disability. The same is true for health-illness dimensions. A person who is healthy because he or she does not
have a disease may still consider himself or herself ill. One
who lacks contentment, or satisfaction with self, others, and
life in general may feel ill, seek health care, and expect treatment. Treatment, however, may not be given. Treatment is
given for a specific disease; if no disease is detected, no medical treatment is given. A person's lack of contentment may
be labeled as a disease. If so, treatment by traditional methods
(drugs, care by a physician, hospitalization) can be given.

Another kind of person could have a diagnosed disease, (e.g., leukemia, cancer, or diabetes) and be healthy from his or her own subjective reference point. Such a person might be healthier than the discontented person just described.

A difficulty of the medical and nursing professions and of society has been evaluation of health-illness from an objective (diagnostic) standpoint rather than from the phenomenological reference point of the individual. Medicine and nursing must focus on the individual's view of his or her own health or illness in order to improve health care. Additional scientific knowledge, research, and practice must help the individual control his or her view of his or her own health. Health care has neglected many variables and interventions that could help a person change his or her behavior or his or her life-style. Correction of the neglect may diminish the frequency and severity of illnesses.

In trying to define health and illness, two types of illnesses appear. One type of illness can easily be diagnosed and treated. The other type is hard to diagnose or define, but it can affect a person more severely than can the first type. Health workers know little about defining and treating the second type of illness. But the second type strongly influences a person's view of his or her own health and therefore affects his or her health.

At a time of struggling with health care and the future concerns and health needs of society, it must be realized that objectivism alone does not hold the solutions to health problems. The traditional "physicalistic" orientation to patient care can no longer be the dominant criterion for health-illness. That view can and must be replaced with a phenomenological view of what health and illness are for each person.

If objective diagnosis and treatment are ineffective in promoting and maintaining health, the health professions, health industries, and society must realize the need for a different emphasis. The different emphasis requires new knowledge and new skill in educating people, promoting or facilitating behavior and life-style change, and helping people to become their own best health care providers.

CHANGING OBSERVATIONS ON AND
EXPLANATIONS FOR ILLNESS

The need for a new and changing emphasis in meeting health care needs is well demonstrated by the epidemic proportions of stress-linked illnesses. Recent findings have linked stress to a variety of mental, physical, and social disorders, among them depression, anxiety, alcoholism, drug addiction, and the breakdown in normal relations with family, friends, and colleagues.

Unrelieved stress can lead to hypertension, coronary disease, migraine-tension headache, peptic ulcer, renal disease, asthma, and even cancer. Stress is also related to social disorders, such as low productivity, absenteeism, divorce, single-parent families, aggression, violence, general dissatisfaction, and illness, hospitalization, and premature death.

In the past, any illness was thought to be caused by a physical agent (e.g., a bacterium). Today, forms of *dis-ease,* such as discontent and worry, are considered illnesses. Forms of *dis-ease,* and many illnesses formerly thought to be caused by physical agents, are now thought to be caused by stress. A person can control the internal or external stress that makes him ill (see Table 11-1).

The discovery that stress can cause illness makes diagnosis and treatment of many illnesses more difficult.

Table 11-1. Changing Explanations of Illness

	In the Past (1900s)	Today (1970s–2000s)
The phenomenon observed	Physical illness	Physical illness or *dis-ease*
Diagnosis/explanation	Illness caused by physical agent (e.g., a bacterium)	Caused by stress; may be cured by self-control and change in life-style

Stress and illnesses caused by stress are more often caused by an individual's life-style, behavior and personality, and social environment than by a bacterium. In the past, physicians always diagnosed the latter and treated their patients for illnesses caused by bacteria rather than by stress.

FACTORS AFFECTING HEALTH: STRESS

Health workers in the future must deal with (1) illnesses
caused by stress-related activities, abuse of substances (food,
alcohol, drugs, cigarettes, air [pollution]) and by interpersonal
support systems (worry, self-concept, self-control), (2) common (acute) illnesses (e.g., upper respiratory tract infection,
vaginitis, gastritis, cancer, hypertension, diabetes, and ortho-
pedic injury), (3) chronic disorders (e.g., ulcers, arthritis,
diabetes, and strokes), and (4) patients before and after hospitalization (to help them recover).

All of the factors just listed are affected by a person's life-
style, personality, behavior, and social environment. In addition to those variables, a person may have physiological
characteristics that make him or her vulnerable to certain
illnesses (e.g., lack of responsiveness of the autonomic nervous
system or of a particular organ system, vulnerability to stress,
lack of stamina, lack of immunity to infection, and existing
illness).

An individual's health may also be related to daily stress and
his or her method of coping with it. The method of coping
may be related to the individual's personality, the plans for one's
life, dreams, and commitments, one's beliefs, goals, and work.
In addition, unresolved developmental conflicts may serve as
hidden agendas in his or her adult life and create special vulnerability. Developmental stages, in which natural transitions occur,
may be full of conflict and promote later stress (e.g., the shifts
from [1] childhood and adolescent dependency to autonomy,
[2] social involvements to intimate relationships, [3] childrearing to the empty nest, and [4] work involvements to retirement).

The association between stress and health can be divided
into the following three broad components: (1) stress inputs,
(2) mediators of stress, and (3) outcomes of stress [30].

Stress Inputs
One major class of inputs that has been well researched is life
changes (see pp. 82–88). Life changes include events such as
the death of a spouse, the loss of a job, a change in residence,
and a vacation. Life changes are of very great importance to

nursing because they affect health. Health maintenance, change, and illness prevention seem to be directly affected by stressful life events and the individual's method of coping with them. The use of a stressful-life-events scale (e.g., the Social Readjustment Rating Scale) in assessing and intervening with health is a unique way to demonstrate a relationship between the biological, psychological, and sociocultural phenomena and health and illness. It appears that an individual who undergoes a great number of life changes in a short period of time undergoes more stress, must cope much more (both psychosocially and biophysically), and is more vulnerable to illness.

Table 11-2 shows the relationship of life changes, life crises, and changes in health.

Table 11-2. Relationship of Life Change Score to Type of Life Crisis

Type of Crisis	Life Change Score (Scores on Social Readjustment Rating Scale)
Mild life crisis	150—199 Life change units
Moderate life crisis	200—299 Life change units
Major life crisis	300+ Life change units

Source: Holmes and Masuda [24].

A moderate number of life crises (scores of 200—299) were often associated with changes in health. The Social Readjustment Rating Scale (see p. 85) is a useful barometer for assessing health and planning intervention to help a patient cope before the fact of illness.

Another kind of stressful input (about which much less is known) is what Lazarus refers to as chronic daily hassles [30, 31]. They include dealing with troubled children, keeping afloat economically, managing unresolved developmental conflicts, managing hostile relationships with peers, colleagues, superiors, and subordinates, and coping with poor marital or family relationships.

A third kind of stress input that affects health and illness is the individual's social environment. The social environment is a system of stimuli that influence the people within the

environment [58]. Many of the ways in which the environment influences an individual are related to the relationships
and support systems in the environment. Other influences
include the milieu, physical setting, esthetics, air, and water.
One's reactions to a clinic waiting room and to hospital environments (such as the intensive care and cardiac care units,
isolation units, and recovery rooms) are also considered stress
inputs.

There is evidence that the family and social environment
may affect recovery and the outcome of therapy. It is well
known that psychological support is closely related to one's
ability to cope and that it promotes impulse control, confidence, extroversion, and decrease in anxiety [58].

The empathy shown by the family of the stroke patient
affects the patient's rate of rehabilitation [43]. Further evidence links poor surgical outcome with high scores on environmental deprivation (including lack of emotional support from
the patient's family) [55].

Other studies have shown that information about the surgery relieves a patient's anxiety and promotes his recovery,
that a supportive relationship and encouragement may supple-
ment care and reduce the length of hospitalization [16, 59].

It appears that the environment can have pronounced positive and negative effects on physiological processes. Such
things as *physical* dimensions (e.g., isolation), *system* dimensions (e.g., orderly, routine work expectations), and *relationship* dimensions can contribute to stress and adversely affect
health. The environmental inputs can affect coping, situational supports, and health improvements.

Mediators of Stress
Regardless of the stress-linked environmental conditions, one's
personal ways of coping with stress can affect the transaction
between the person and the environment. One's way of coping is reported to be influenced by at least four factors: (1) the
degree of uncertainty perceived, (2) the degree of threat,
(3) the presence of conflict, and (4) the degree of helplessness
[30]. Thus the effect of environmental inputs on the stress-
health related outcomes depends on a variety of psychological

and physiological processes, including the way the individual *perceives* the environmental demands and the *patterns* of coping he or she employs to master a stressful situation [30].

Given the same social environmental inputs, different kinds of people may perceive different degrees of uncertainty, threat, conflict, or helplessness. An insecure, suspicious person may perceive that he has little support, few options, and little internal control. Likewise, different kinds of people may differ in their adapting or coping responses, depending on their perceptions and personalities. One person may be confident and assertive in manipulating his environment; another person may withdraw, give up, and feel defeated.

Another mediator of stress that is related to the person's perception of environmental input is his personality, as shown most clearly by the Type A personality work of Rosenman and Friedman [44]. A person who is consumed with a sense of the importance of time and deadlines and who is aggressive and competitive is more apt to suffer ill health from stress than is someone who moves at a slower pace and can relax and enjoy diversions.

The correlation of personality type and cancer has been studied by different groups in different countries. A consistent picture emerges. A variety of objective and projective questionnaires and tests show that the typical cancer patient is a rigid, authoritarian, inner-directed, and religious person who has conflicts about sex and hostility and poor emotional outlets. He or she uses excessive repression to handle his or her emotions [48]. (See also the works of Bahnson and co-workers [6, 7], Cobb [13], Le Shan [34], Le Shan and co-workers [33, 35], and Reznikoff [42].)

Studies of the causes of cancers have found that the following two kinds of stress-response personalities promote the development of cancer:

1. A repressive personality that is affected by specific experiences in childhood
2. A personality that responds with hopelessness-helplessness-despair to a life situation or the loss of a significant other.

A third class of stress mediators associated with methods of coping and illness caused by stress are behaviors associated with a person's feeling of control or of helplessness. A person's choice of a method of coping with a problem depends on whether he feels that he has any control over the problem. A series of psychological experiments have centered on perceived control [22]. A feeling of control mediates between the stressful input and the effect of stress on health. A person's sense of control (or lack of control) is part of his self-appraisal. Studies have explored both generalized expectations and specific expectations of people pursuing particular goals. "Results from both types of studies conclude that the manner in which individuals appraise themselves with regard to causality makes a difference in the way that many life experiences will be confronted [32]." Factors that mediate stress, such as personality type and feeling of control, should be considered by nurses who are planning interventions.

Outcomes of Stress
Stress-related outcomes are associated with a person's health-illness and work-social functioning and morale. A wide variety of health conditions have been linked to stress. They range from mental depression to physiological disorders (e.g., cancer) to work problems (e.g., absenteeism). In assessing the effects of stress on health, many dimensions of functioning should be considered — the individual's functioning in society and at work and his mental state, as well as his health.

The broad effects of stress on health are now discussed in terms of wellness. The idea of assessing wellness and promoting high levels of wellness through stress-coping interventions is relatively new. Recently, the Wellness Inventory was devised (see Table 11-3). Both the nurse and health consumer can use that scale to help a person see himself or herself as a growing, changing person who needs to take good care of himself or herself. The Wellness Inventory can teach someone to use his mind constructively, to express his emotions effectively, to be creatively involved with others, to be concerned about his physical and psychological environments, and to become aware

Table 11-3. Wellness Inventory

INSTRUCTIONS

Please put a mark in the box before each statement which is true *for you*. Total each section, then copy the subtotals to the back page. Average total scores range from 65 to 75. (If you are answering this questionnaire as part of a wellness evaluation, when the evaluation is completed, this copy of the booklet will be given to you for future reference.)

WHAT IS MEANT BY WELLNESS?

The ideas of measuring wellness and helping people attain high levels of wellness are relatively new. Most of us think in terms of illness and assume that the absence of illness indicates wellness. This is not true. There are many degrees of wellness as there are many degrees of illness. The diagram below is a model used by well medicine.

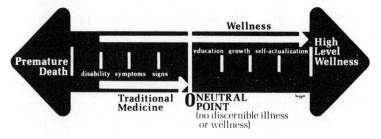

Moving from the center to the left shows a progressively worsening state of health. Moving to the right of center shows increasing levels of health and well-being. Traditional medicine is oriented towards curing evidence of disease, but usually stops at the midpoint. Well medicine begins at any point on the scale with the goal of helping a person to move as far to the right as possible.

Many people lack physical symptoms but are bored, depressed, tense, anxious or generally unhappy with their lives. These emotional states often lead to physical disease through the lowering of the body's resistance. The same feelings can also lead to abuse of the body through smoking, drinking and overeating. These behaviors are usually substitutes for other more basic human needs such as recognition from others, a stimulating environment, caring and affection from friends, and growth towards higher levels of self-awareness.

Wellness is not a static state. It results when a person begins to see himself as a growing, changing person. High level wellness means giving good care to your physical self, using your mind constructively, expressing your emotions effectively, being creatively involved with those around you, being concerned about your physical and psychological environment and becoming aware of other levels of consciousness.

This questionnaire will help to give you an idea about where you presently are on the wellness scale.

1. *Productivity, Relaxation, Sleep*

00 ☐ I usually enjoy my work.
01 ☐ I seldom feel tired and rundown (except after strenuous work).*
02 ☐ I fall asleep easily at bedtime.
03 ☐ I usually get a full night's sleep.
04 ☐ If awakened, it is usually easy for me to go to sleep again.
05 ☐ I rarely bite or pick at my nails.
06 ☐ Rather than worrying, I can temporarily shelve my problems and enjoy myself at times when I can do nothing about solving them immediately.
07 ☐ I feel financially secure.
08 ☐ I am content with my sexual life.
09 ☐ I meditate or center myself for 15 to 20 minutes at least once a day.*

☐
Total
Checked

2. *Personal Care and Home Safety*

10 ☐ I take measures to protect my living space from fire and safety hazards (such as improper sized fuses and storage of volatile chemicals).
11 ☐ I have a dry chemical fire extinguisher in my kitchen and at least one other extinguisher elsewhere in my living quarters. (If very small apartment, kitchen extinguisher alone is adequate).*
12 ☐ I regularly use dental floss and a soft toothbrush.*
13 ☐ I smoke less than one pack of cigarettes or equivalent cigars or pipes *per week*.
14 ☐ I don't smoke at all (if this statement is true, mark item above true as well).
15 ☐ I keep an up-to-date record of my immunizations.
16 ☐ I have fewer than three colds per year.*
17 ☐ I minimize my exposure to sprays, chemical fumes or exhaust gases.*
18 ☐ I avoid extremely noisy areas (or wear protective ear plugs).*
19 ☐ I am aware of changes in my physical or mental state and seek professional advice about any which seem unusual.

Women

100 ☐ I check my breasts for unusual lumps once a month.
101 ☐ I have a pap test annually.

Men

☐
Total
Checked

102 ☐ If uncircumcised, I am aware of the special need for regular cleansing under my foreskin.
103 ☐ If over 45, I have my prostate checked annually.

* An asterisk at the end of a statement indicates that there is a footnote for that statement on the last page.

3. *Nutritional Awareness*

20 ☐ I eat at least one uncooked fruit or vegetable each day.*
21 ☐ I have fewer than three alcoholic drinks (including beer) per week.
22 ☐ I rarely take medications, including prescription drugs.
23 ☐ I drink fewer than five soft drinks per week.*
24 ☐ I avoid eating refined foods or foods with sugar added.
25 ☐ I add little salt to my food.*
26 ☐ I read the labels for the ingredients of the foods I buy.
27 ☐ I add unprocessed bran to my diet to provide roughage.*
28 ☐ I drink fewer than three cups of coffee or tea (with the exception of herbal teas)
       a day.*
29 ☐ I have a good appetite and maintain a weight within 15% of my ideal weight.

☐
Total
Checked

4. *Environmental Awareness*

30 ☐ I use public transportation or car pools when possible.
31 ☐ I turn off unneeded lights or appliances.
32 ☐ I recycle papers, cans, glass, clothing, books and organic waste (mark true if
       you do at least three of these).
33 ☐ I set my thermostat at 68° or lower in winter.
34 ☐ I use air conditioning only when necessary and keep the thermostat at 76°
       or higher.
35 ☐ I am conscientious about wasted energy and materials both at home and at work.
36 ☐ I use nonpolluting cleaning agents.
37 ☐ My car gets at least 18 miles per gallon. (If you don't own a car, check this
       statement as true).
38 ☐ I have storm windows and adequate insulation in attic and walls. (If you don't
       own your home or live in a mild climate, check this statement as true).
39 ☐ I have a humidifier for use in winter. (If you don't have central heating check this
       statement as true).*

☐
Total
Checked

5. *Physical Activity*

40 ☐ I climb stairs rather than ride elevators.
41 ☐ My daily activities include moderate physical effort (such as rearing young
       children, gardening, scrubbing floors, or work which involves being on my feet,
       etc.).
42 ☐ My daily activities include vigorous physical effort (such as heavy construction
       work, farming, moving heavy objects by hand, etc.).
43 ☐ I run at least one mile twice a week (or equivalent aerobic exercise).*
44 ☐ I run at least one mile four times a week or equivalent (if this statement is true,
       mark the item above true as well).*
45 ☐ I regularly walk or ride a bike for exercise.
46 ☐ I participate in a strenuous sport at least once a week.
47 ☐ I participate in a strenuous sport more than once a week (if this statement is
       true, mark the item above true as well).
48 ☐ I do yoga or some form of stretching-limbering exercise for 15 to 20 minutes at
       least twice per week.*
49 ☐ I do yoga or some form of stretching exercise for 15 to 20 minutes at least
       four times per week (if this statement is true, mark the item above true as well).

☐
Total
Checked

6. *Expression of Emotions and Feelings*

50 ☐ I am frequently happy.
51 ☐ I think it is OK to feel angry, afraid, joyful or sad.*
52 ☐ I do not deny my anger, fear, joy or sadness, but instead find constructive ways to express these feelings most of the time.*
53 ☐ I am able to say "no" to people without feeling guilty.
54 ☐ It is easy for me to laugh.
55 ☐ I like getting compliments and recognition from other people.
56 ☐ I feel OK about crying, and allow myself to do so.*
57 ☐ I listen to and think about constructive criticism rather than react defensively.
58 ☐ I would seek help from friends or professional counselors if needed.
59 ☐ It is easy for me to give other people sincere compliments and recognition.

☐
Total
Checked

7. *Community Involvement*

60 ☐ I keep informed of local, national and world events.
61 ☐ I vote regularly.
62 ☐ I take interest in community, national and world events and work to support issues and people of my choice. (If this statement is true, mark both items above true as well.)
63 ☐ When I am able, I contribute time or money to worthy causes.
64 ☐ I make an attempt to know my neighbors and be on good terms with them.
65 ☐ If I saw a crime being committed, I would call the police.
66 ☐ If I saw a broken bottle lying in the road or on the sidewalk, I would remove it.
67 ☐ When driving, I am considerate of pedestrians and other drivers.
68 ☐ If I saw a car with faulty lights, leaking gasoline or another dangerous condition, I would attempt to inform the driver.
69 ☐ I am a member of one or more community organizations (social change group, singing group, club, church or political group).

☐
Total
Checked

8. *Creativity, Self Expression*

70 ☐ I enjoy expressing myself through art, dance, music, drama, sports, etc.
71 ☐ I enjoy spending some time without planned or structured activities.*
72 ☐ I usually meet several people a month who I would like to get to know better.
73 ☐ I enjoy touching other people.*
74 ☐ I enjoy being touched by other people.*
75 ☐ I have at least five close friends.
76 ☐ At times I like to be alone.
77 ☐ I like myself and look forward to the future.
78 ☐ I look forward to living to be at least 75.*
79 ☐ I find it easy to express concern, love and warmth to those I care about.

☐
Total
Checked

9. *Automobile Safety*

If you don't own an automobile and ride less than 1,000 miles per year in one, enter 7 points in the box at left and skip the next 10 questions. (If you ride more than 1,000 miles per year but don't own a car, answer as many statements as you can and show this copy to the car's owner.)

80 ☐ I never drink when driving.
81 ☐ I wear a lap safety belt at least 90% of the time that I ride in a car.*
81a ☐ I wear a shoulder-lap belt at least 90% of the time that I ride in a car. (If this statement is true, mark the item above true as well.)*
82 ☐ I stay within 5 mph of the speed limit.
83 ☐ My car has head restraints on the front seats and I keep them adjusted high enough to protect myself and passengers from whiplash injuries.*
84 ☐ I frequently inspect my automobile tires, lights, etc. and have my car serviced regularly.
85 ☐ I have disc brakes on my car.*
86 ☐ I drive on belted radial tires.*
87 ☐ I carry emergency flares or reflectors and a fire extinguisher in my car.
88 ☐ I stop on yellow when a traffic light is changing.
89 ☐ For every 10 mph of speed, I maintain a car length's distance from the car ahead of me.

☐
Total
Checked

10. *Parenting*

If you don't have any responsibility for young children, enter 7 in the box at left and skip the next 10 questions. (If some of the questions are not applicable because your children are no longer young, answer them as you would if they were youngsters again.)

90 ☐ When riding in a car, I make certain that any child weighing under 50 pounds is secured in an approved child's safety seat or safety harness similar to those sold by the major auto manufacturers.*
91 ☐ When riding in a car, I make certain that any child weighing over 50 pounds is wearing an adult seat belt/shoulder harness.*
92 ☐ When leaving my child(ren), I make certain that the person in charge has the telephone numbers of my pediatrician or a hospital for emergency use.
93 ☐ I don't let my children ride escalators in bare feet or tennis shoes.*
94 ☐ I do not store cleaning products under the sink or in unlocked cabinets where a child could reach them.
95 ☐ I have a lock on the medicine cabinet or other places where medicines are stored.
96 ☐ I prepare my own baby food with a baby food grinder—thus avoiding commercial foods.*
97 ☐ I have sought information on parenting and raising children.
98 ☐ I frequently touch or hold my children.
99 ☐ I respect my child as an evolving, growing being.

☐
Total
Checked

ENTER SUBTOTALS ON BACK COVER

FOOTNOTES

Numbers before each statement refer to a statement above. Numbers following statements indicate references (next page).

01. Fatigue without apparent cause is not a normal condition and usually indicates illness, stress or denial of emotional expression. (14)
09. Meditation or centering greatly enhances one's sense of well being. (1, 2, 12, 13)
11. Many injuries and much damage can be prevented by putting out fires when they first start. Dry chemical or CO_2 fire extinguishers are necessary for oil, grease and electrical fires.
12. Regular flossing and using a good soft toothbrush with rounded tip bristles prevent the premature loss of teeth in one's 40s and 50s. Be sure to learn the proper techniques of use from a dental hygienist or dentist. (3)
16. If you have more than three colds a year, you may not be getting enough rest, eating a good diet or meeting other energy needs properly. (4)
17. All such toxins have a harmful effect on the liver and other tissues over long periods of time.
18. Very loud noises which leave your ears ringing can cause permanent hearing loss which accumulates and is usually not noticeable until one reaches 40 or 50. Small cushioned ear plugs (not the type designed for swimmers), wax ear plugs and accoustic ear muffs (which look like stereo headphones without wires) can often be purchased in sporting goods stores.
20. Fresh fruits and vegetables provide vitamins, minerals, trace nutrients and roughage which are often lacking in modern diets. (5, 11)
23. Soft drinks are high in refined sugar which provides only "empty" calories and usually replace foods which have more nutritional value. Artificially sweetened soft drinks consumed in excess may have long-range consequences as yet not known. (Both types of soft drinks contain caffeine or other stimulants.)
25. Salting foods during cooking draws many vitamins out of the food and into the water which is usually discarded. Heavy salting of foods at the table may cause a strain on the kidneys and result in high blood pressure. (4)
27. Wheat bran, usually removed in the commercial milling of wheat, is the single best source of dietary fiber available. The use of approximately two tablespoons per day (individual needs vary) can substantially reduce colon cancer, diverticulosis, heart disease and other conditions related to refined food diets.
28. Coffee and tea (other than herbal teas) contain stimulants which, if abused, do not allow one's body to function normally. (4)
ENVIRONMENTAL AWARENESS. Taking care of your environment affects your own wellness as well as everyone else's.
39. Humidified heated air allows one to set the thermostat several degrees lower and still feel as warm as without humidification. It also helps prevent many respiratory ailments. House plants will require less watering and will be happier too.
43, 44. Vigorous aerobic exercise (such as running) must keep the heart rate at 150 beats per minute for 12 to 20 minutes to produce the "training effect." Less vigorous aerobic exercise (lower heart rate) must be maintained for much longer periods to produce the same benefit. The "training effect" is necessary to prepare the heart for meeting extra strain. (6)
48. Such exercise prevents stiffness of joints and musculo-skeletal degeneration. It also promotes a greater feeling of well-being. (7)
51. Basic emotions, if repressed, often cause anxiety, depression, irrational behavior or physical disease. People can relearn to feel and express their emotions with a resulting improvement in their well-being. Some people, however, exaggerate emotions to control and manipulate others; tnis can be detrimental to their well-being. (8, 9)
52. Learning ways to constructively express these emotions (so that all parties concerned feel better) leads to more satisfying relationships and problem solving. (8, 9)
56. Crying over a loss or sad event is an important discharge of emotional energy. It is, however, sometimes used as a manipulative tool, or as a substitute expression of anger. Many males in particular have been erroneously taught that it is not OK to cry. (8)

FOOTNOTES (cont'd)

71. Spending time spontaneously without relying on an external structure can be self-renewing. (8)
73, 74. Physical touch is important for the maintenance of life for young children and remains important throughout adult life. (10)
78. With proper self care, most individuals can easily reach this age in good health.
81. Shoulder/lap belts are much safer than lap belts alone. (Shoulder belts should never be worn without a lap belt.)
83. Whiplash injuries can be prevented by properly adjusted head restraints. These are required, in the U.S., on the front seats of all autos made since 1968 but are often not raised high enough to protect passengers and driver.
85. Disc brakes provide considerably better braking power than conventional drum brakes.
86. For most cars, radial tires maintain firmer contact with the road and improve braking and handling better than bias ply tires. They also have less rolling friction and give better gas mileage.
90, 91. Over 1,000 young children a year are killed in motor vehicle accidents in the U.S. Many deaths can be prevented by keeping the child from flying about in a car crash. Most car seats do not provide enough protection—as government standards are very low. Check consumer magazines for up-to-date information. Never use an adult seat belt for a child weighing less than 50 pounds.
93. The bare feet of young children are often injured at the end of escalators. Wearing tennis shoes is equally dangerous because their sturdy long laces get pulled into the mechanism and their thin canvas walls offer little protection.
96. Commercial baby foods contain high amounts of sugar, salt, modified starches and preservatives which may adversely affect a baby's future eating habits and health. Federal legislation has been introduced to help correct this problem. Portable baby food grinders and blenders can be used to prepare for an infant the same food as eaten by the rest of the family. Individual servings can be packaged and frozen for future meals.

SCORING

Enter subtotals from each section below and compute your total score.

1 ☐ Productivity
2 ☐ Care & Safety
3 ☐ Nutrition
4 ☐ Environment
5 ☐ Physical
6 ☐ Emotions
7 ☐ Community
8 ☐ Creativity
9 ☐ Auto
10 ☐ Parenting

Total _____

REFERENCES

1. *Human Life Styling* - McCamy
2. *Be Here Now* - Ram Dass
3. *The Tooth Trip* - McGuire
4. *Well Body Book* - Samuels and Bennett
5. *Nutrition Against Disease* - Williams
6. *The New Aerobics* and *Aerobics for Women* - Cooper
7. *Fundamentals of Yoga* - Mishra
8. *Born to Win* - James and Jongeward
9. *The Angry Book* - Rubin
10. *Touching* - Montague
11. *Diet for a Small Planet* - Lappe
12. *Center of the Cyclone* - Lilly
13. *The Crack in the Cosmic Egg* - Pearce
14. *Stress* - McQuade & Aiken

of other levels of consciousness. Such a scale can be a useful intervention tool for both consumers and nurses who are concerned with health in its broadest sense.

It appears that today the following things are happening simultaneously to accommodate the new knowledge and change the health scene:

1. Medicine is moving away from a traditional medical model toward holistic care, a trend that is reflected in the fact that medical schools teach the social and behavioral sciences and offer an increase in primary care in family practice options.
2. Nursing also is expanding its already comprehensive position to a fully developed, autonomous position that emphasizes holistic self-care and high levels of wellness. That trend is reflected by the increasing numbers of nurses in private practice, the focus on wellness and continuity of care, and the emphasis on teaching, counseling, and psychosocial intervention.
3. Lay and Self-help groups have served as support systems for millions of people that have needs to which health care systems do not address themselves (e.g., single-parent groups, battered-partners groups, overeaters groups, lay midwives, and childbirth educators).
4. Alternative health care systems have developed to change the traditional medical model.

The Association for Healing Arts and the Association for Holistic Health are examples of groups that attempt to merge health care with people's day-to-day lives. Many of the alternative approaches to health care advocate self-control through a broad spectrum of theories and practices. They encourage a person to concern himself or herself with the environment (e.g., to fight pollution of air and water), and nutrition (e.g., to live on a macrobiotic diet), and to use special therapies (e.g., acupuncture, biofeedback, hypnosis, and autogenic control).

Some of those concerns are incorporated into traditional medical and nursing care practice. For example, an increasing number of clinicians use mind control, biofeedback, and meditation to accompany traditional Western medical treatment. Some of those practices have helped people suffering from hypertension, migraine headache, chronic pain, and even cancer. It has been speculated that people who incorporate self-control into their lives and modify their high-stress life-styles may be healthier and have fewer physiological disorders than have people who do not control themselves and their life-styles.

The changing health needs of society, combined with an increased consumer awareness and activity, have changed the health professionals' orientation to health and illness. In the future, health professionals must give the patient responsibility and self-control so that he or she can assume self-care. They must teach the patient (and his or her family) how to cope with stress. Such an approach focuses care on the patient and (or) his or her family as a unit. More than ever before, holistic health care must promote a higher quality of life and help people direct their mental and physical energies in order to deal more effectively with stress.

The changing focus of health care requires expanded knowledge and skill and an expanded human value system in regard to (1) a higher quality of life, (2) the ability to face one's limits and adjust to them, (3) the capacity to understand one's successes and failures, and (4) a philosophy that enables one to cope with the inevitable emotional crises of life, such as caring for another person, or facing death (either one's own or that of a loved one). The new health care is guided by science and humanism, and it has the orientation and patience that allow and support a person's own healing processes.

Basic humanistic values and psychosocial knowledge often determine the degree to which the nurse is able to understand the patient's growth and adaptive and maladaptive behavior, to help the patient use all his or her potential, and to help the patient find the highest quality of life possible for him or her. All those variables may ultimately define health since health in its broadest sense is high-quality *living*. Major breakthroughs may be required before health professionals are able to view their role as one of helping people to *live* fully. It may be the *caring*

focus that will allow nurses to contribute the most to the
health of a people and a society.

RECENT PROFESSIONAL DIRECTIONS
Nursing is making significant gains in accommodating itself to
the health needs of society. The American Academy of Nursing was established in 1973 to:

1. Advance new concepts in health care
2. Identify and explore issues in health, in the health profes-
    sions, and in society (as those issues affect and are affected
    by nurses and nursing)
3. Examine the dynamics of nursing, the interrelationships of
    the divisions of nursing, and to examine the interactions
    among nurses (as all those factors affect the development
    of nursing)
4. Identify and propose resolutions to issues and problems
    confronting nursing and health, including alternative plans
    for implementation [4]

The growing emphasis in nursing on primary care and higher
levels of education has produced nurses who can accept responsibility for their health care practice and who are accountable
for their actions to their clients and society.
U.S. society has had an evolving health care delivery system
in which the health services are not equitably distributed.
Health care is often fragmented and uncoordinated, and it
often does not address itself to human needs. Health care
often discourages people from participating in their own
health care. Inefficient, expensive, "after-the-fact" medical
treatment is substituted for health care. However, the health
care delivery system in the United States is changing to reflect
changing views of health. Nursing plays a major role in the
change. More consumer input makes health care emphasize
health behaviors, life-style, and coping. Both the nursing and
medical professions and the health industries recognize the
need to improve the health care delivery system in regard to
quality, availability, continuity, and cost-effectiveness.

As the concerns of and changes in nursing develop, more and more nurses are being prepared to assume major responsibilities in health care. Recent findings provide some evidence regarding the significant role nurses can play in solving some of the health care problems. The evidence supports the important role of nurses' health care delivery now and in the future [36].

SUMMARY

This chapter has developed the concept of health in the broad sense that health is a dynamic process in which a person moves forward and upward toward a higher level of functioning. Nursing as the science of caring is especially oriented toward maximizing the holistic health potential of the individual and the family. The health care provider has learned that recent changes in health care delivery have given individuals and families the power to decide about the quality of their health and health care. The new emphasis on self-care and self-control is regarded as necessary for high-quality health. Health professionals now readily agree that the individual and his or her family are the best providers of health care. The self-control that an individual can use to cope and adapt to stress is now recognized as a valuable mediating process. New knowledge about the effect of stress inputs from one's environment and other mediating forces (such as one's personality, perception of environmental stimuli, and degree of control over one's environment) on one's health help to promote health.

If health-wellness is the concept that guides the practice of nursing and the science of caring, new, nonmedical models must be continually explored. This chapter discussed some of the major health forces that must be considered for the practice of the science of caring.

REFERENCES

1. Allen, T. W. Physical Health. *Personnel and Guidance Journal* 56:40, 1977.
2. American Academy of Nursing. Primary Care by Nurses: Sphere of Responsibility and Accountability. Kansas City, Mo.: American Academy of Nursing, 1977. Pp. 1–2.

3. Angle, M., and Walters, R. AMA Doesn't Learn Very Well. *Rocky Mountain News,* Denver (Colorado), July 21, 1977. P. 56.

4. Appley, M. H., and Trumbull, R. *Psychological Stress.* New York: Appleton-Century-Crofts, 1967.

5. Bahnson, C. B. (ed.). Second conference on psychophysiological aspects of cancer. *Annals of the New York Academy of Science* 164:307, 1969.

6. Bahnson, C. B., and Bahnson, M. B. Role of ego defenses: Denial and repression in the etiology of malignant neoplasm. *Annals of the New York Academy of Science* 125:827, 1966.

7. Bahnson, C. B., and Kissen, D. M. (eds.). Psychophysiological aspects of cancer. *Annals of the New York Academy of Science* 125:773, 1966.

8. Bahnson, M. B., and Bahnson, C. B. Ego defenses in cancer patients. *Annals of the New York Academy of Science* 164:546, 1969.

9. Beecher, H. K. Quantification of the Subjective Pain Experience. In P. H. Hoch and J. Zubin (eds.), *Psychopathology of Perception.* New York: Grune & Stratton, 1965. Pp. 111–128.

10. Benson, H. *The Relaxation Response.* New York: Morrow, 1975.

11. Burns, E. M. *Health Services for Tomorrow: Trends and Issues.* New York: Dunellen, 1973.

12. Cannon, W. B. Recent studies of bodily effects of fear, rage, and pain. *Journal of Philosophy, Psychology and Scientific Methods* 11:162, 1914.

13. Cobb, B. Emotional problems of adult cancer patients. *Journal of the American Geriatric Society* 1:274, 1959.

14. Coelho, G. V., Hamburg, D. A., and Adams, J. E. (eds.). *Coping and Adaptation.* New York: Basic Books, 1974.

15. Dohrenwend, B. S., and Dohrenwend, B. P. (eds.). *Stressful Life Events.* New York: Wiley, 1974.

16. Egbert, L., Battit, G., Welch, C., et al. Reduction of postoperative pain by encouragement and instruction of patients. *New England Journal of Medicine* 270:825, 1964.

17. Engel, G. L. Too little science: The paradox in modern medicine's crisis. *Pharos* 39:127, 1976.

18. Engel, G. L. *Psychological Development in Health and Disease.* Philadelphia: Saunders, 1963.

19. Fox, R. The medicalization and demedicalization of American society. *Daedalus: Journal of the American Academy of Arts and Sciences* 106:9, 1977.

20. Friedman, M., and Rosenman, R. G. *Type A Behavior and Your Heart.* Greenwich, Conn.: Crest Books (Fawcett), 1975.

21. Geyman, J. P. Is there a difference between nursing practice and medical practice. *Journal of Family Practice* 5:935, 1977.

22. Glass, D. C., and Singer, J. E. *Urban Stress.* New York: Academic, 1972.

23. Greene, W. A. The psychological setting of the development of leukemia and lymphoma. *Annals of the New York Academy of Science* 125:794, 1966.
24. Holmes, T. H., and Masuda, M. Life Change and Illness Susceptibility. In B. S. Dohrenwend and B. P. Dohrenwend (eds.), *Stressful Life Events.* New York: Wiley, 1974. Pp. 45–72.
25. Illich, I. *Medical Nemesis.* New York: Pantheon Books (Random House), 1976.
26. Janis, I. *Psychological Stress.* New York: Wiley, 1958.
27. Jenkins, C. D. Psychologic and social precursors of coronary disease. *New England Journal of Medicine* 284:224, 307, 1971.
28. Jenkins, C. D., et al. Prediction of clinical coronary heart disease by a test of the coronary-prone behavior pattern. *New England Journal of Medicine* 290:3, 1974.
29. Knowles, J. H. Introduction. *Daedalus: Journal of the American Academy of Arts and Sciences* 106:1, 1977.
30. Lazarus, R. S., and Cohen, J. B. Theory and Method in the Study of Stress and Coping in Aging Individuals. Paper read in June, 1976, at the Fifth World Health Organization Conference on Society, Stress and Disease held in Stockholm, Sweden. New York: Oxford University Press. In press.
31. Lazarus, R., and Launier, R. Stress-related Transactions Between Person and Environment. In L. A. Pervin and M. Lewis (eds.), *Internal and External Determinants of Behavior.* New York: Plenum, 1978.
32. Lefcourt, H. M. *Locus of Control.* New York: Wiley, 1976. P. 141.
33. Le Shan, L. L. An emotional life-history pattern associated with neoplastic disease. *Annals of the New York Academy of Science* 125:780, 1966.
34. Le Shan, L. L., and Reznikoff, M. A. Psychological factors apparently associated with neoplastic disease. *Journal of Abnormal Soc. Psych.* 60:439, 1960.
35. Le Shan, L. L., and Worthington, R. E. Some recurrent life history patterns observed in patients with malignant disease. *Journal of Nervous and Mental Disease* 124:460, 1956.
36. Levine, E. What do we know about nurse practitioners? *American Journal of Nursing* 77:1799, 1977.
37. Lipkin, M. *The Care of Patients.* New York: Oxford University Press, 1974.
38. Moos, R. *The Human Context: Environmental Determinants of Behavior.* New York: Wiley, 1976.
39. Nimetz, M. Report of a Symposium. In Andreopoulos Spyros (ed.), *Primary Care: Where Medicine Fails.* New York: Wiley, 1974. Pp. 187–199.
40. Pelletier, K. R. *Mind As Healer, Mind As Slayer.* New York: Dell, 1977.

41. Rahe, R. H. The Pathway Between Subjects' Recent Life Changes and Their Near Future Illness Reports. In B. S. Dohrenwend and B. P. Dohrenwend (eds.), *Stressful Life Events*. New York: Wiley, 1974. Pp. 73–86.
42. Reznikoff, N. Psychological factors in breast cancer. *Psychosomatic Medicine* 17:96, 1955.
43. Robertson, E., and Suinn, R. The determination of the rate of progress of stroke patients through empathy measure of patient and family. *Journal of Psychosomatic Research* 12:189, 1968.
44. Rosenman, R. H., and Friedman, M. The Central Nervous System and Coronary Heart Disease. In P. Insel, and R. Moos (eds.), *Health and the Social Environment*. Lexington, Mass.: Health, 1974. Pp. 93–100.
45. Rozak, T. Letter to the editor. *Science* 187:790, 1975.
46. Schmale, A. H. Relations of separation and depression to disease. *Psychosomatic Medicine* 20:259, 1958.
47. Schmale, A. H. Needs, gratifications and the vicissitudes of the self representation. *Psychoanalytic Study of Society* 2:9, 1962.
48. Schofield, W., Bahnson, C., Hardee, B., Kelty, E., et al. A.P.A. Task Force on Health Research. Contributions of Psychology to Health Research: Patterns, Problems and Potentials. Unpublished manuscript, 1977.
49. Seligman, M. E. P. *Helplessness*. San Francisco: Freeman, 1975.
50. Selye, H. *The Stress of Life*. New York: McGraw-Hill, 1956.
51. Smith, A. *Powers of the Mind*. New York: Random House, 1975.
52. Soloman, G. F. Emotion, stress and the central nervous system, and immunity. *Annals of the New York Academy of Science* 164:335, 1969.
53. Soloman, G. F., Amkraut, A. A., and Kasper, P. Immunity, emotions and stress. *Journal of Psychotherapy and Psychosomatics* 23:29, 1974.
54. Tanner, O., et al. *Stress*. New York: Time-Life Books, 1976.
55. Throughman, J., Pascal, G., Jarvis, J., and Crutcher, J. A study of psychological factors in patients with surgically intractable duodenal ulcers and those with other intractable disorders. *Psychosomatic Medicine* 29:273, 1967.
56. Travis, J. W. Wellness Scale. Mill Valley, Calif.: Wellness Resource Center, 1977.
57. Wildavsky, A. Doing better and feeling worse. *Daedalus: Journal of the American Academy of Arts and Sciences*. 106:105, 1977.
58. Wittkower, E. D., and Warnes, H. (eds.). *Psychosomatic Medicine*. New York: Harper & Row, 1977.
59. Wolf, R. The Measurement of Environments. In A. Anastasi (ed.), *Testing Problems in Perspective*. Washington, D.C.: American Council on Education, 1966.
60. Wolff, H. G. *Stress and Disease*. Springfield, Ill.: Thomas, 1953.
61. Zubek, John P. (ed.). *Sensory Deprivation: Fifteen Years of Research*. New York: Appleton-Century-Crofts, 1969.

12. DEVELOPMENTAL CONFLICTS

A common condition and a normal life process that is believed to be important from a standpoint of intervention-knowledge for health and the practice of care is the phenomenon of *developmental conflicts.* Chapter 12 explains the developmental conflicts of the individual and the family as common, normal life processes that can affect one's ability to cope with the stress of health-illness and that may be the bases for generating stress that requires a coping response.

Each phase of growth and development brings with it conflicts and growth issues that affect one's present and future development and health. Unresolved conflicts of development left over from one's childhood may serve as hidden agendas in one's adult life. Certain vulnerabilities can be created by normal transitions in development and contribute to stress in the present and future. Such transitions include the shift from dependence of childhood to adolescent and young-adult goals of independence or the shift from one level of functioning to another, such as from the work-social level to the personal-sexual level — and vice versa.

One health goal is the promotion of the individual's growth to the highest level possible. As nurses come to understand the life cycle, they can more effectively plan, intervene, and evaluate the supportive, adaptive, and growth behaviors that improve the quality of a patient's life. A large part of an individual's development during his life is psychosocial. Psychosocial development stimulates self-actualization, or the resolution of developmental conflicts.

Human behavior changes constantly throughout life. It has both biological and psychosocial factors that work interdependently to produce behavioral development. A person is never without an environment or a biological system that affects his or her behavior. However, the psychosocial aspects of human development are the most neglected ones, especially from the adolescent years to old age. Each stage brings special psychosocial conflicts and developmental problems.

INDIVIDUAL DEVELOPMENTAL CONFLICTS

Erikson referred to the separate developmental phases as crises. The individual must overcome each crisis at the proper time and in the proper sequence.

In Erikson's view, developmental conflicts and crises are normal and growth producing for each person provided the proper resources and coping and support systems for the crises are available when the person confronts the crisis. Development is thus inherently tied to health and holistic care.

A human growth and developmental conflicts model assumes that regression is normal and even necessary for future growth. It is also probable that whenever a person responds to and copes with intense internal or external stress-change, loss, or illness, he will regress. The regression to previous developmental phases is considered to be a natural one. Then, developmental crises that were previously surmounted are reworked. Regression coincides with psychological turning points. The conflict at turning points is between (1) progress and regression and (2) integration and retardation.

Developmental psychologists theorize that each phase of development is correlated with a critical psychological-social task that must be accomplished regardless of the biological maturation and growth process. The psychosocial task accomplishments and intervention behaviors for holistic care include some assessment and attempts to understand the developmental conflicts and needs of the parents, as well as the developmental conflicts and needs of their child. Systematic attention to developmental conflicts of individuals and their families is necessary for health care. One area into which nursing must move — in terms of furthering knowledge and developing effective interventions — is stress. The other area is developmental conflict. The nurse needs not only basic knowledge but also assertiveness in assessing and intervening with developmental conflicts in order to provide holistic health care. The nurse must also be aware of the phenomena of regression and retardation and of the reworking process in order to help the person integrate his developmental tasks.

The reworking is a dynamic process that involves everyone from birth to death. If health is to be affected, primary nursing

care related to growth and development must be systematically attentive to the more subtle and inner changes that are
operating psychodynamically and psychosocially in a person's
life as well as to the biophysical changes that accompany
chronological development. It is somewhat understandable
that nursing has been ambivalent in its assertiveness or commitment to that area. Theories of child development have
changed in the course of time. Even though some theories
have become established, people tend to hold to their own
theories, which are often important determinants for parental
action and perhaps professional action.

In order to consider a child's psychosocial development, a
nurse must consider the child's case and health histories, the
verbal and nonverbal communication between parents and
child, observation of the child, and an interview with the
child's parents about the child. The systematic counseling
begins with pregnancy and parent-infant bonding, continues
into later childhood and adolescence, and on into young adulthood, maturity, and old age.

Each of these life phases brings with it particular psychosocial developmental problems that the person tests out, reex-
amines, reworks, and resolves. Each phase can be a critical
determinant of how subsequent development will proceed.
Each phase can be a turning point toward growth or illness.
Each person struggles to some degree with his or her own psychosocial conflicts, identity, and intactness in every phase of
development. If the struggle does not occur and the issues are
not confronted, the psychological maturing ability of the person can be retarded. As one "grows up" psychologically and
chronologically, the personality faces "hazards of existence
continuously, even as the body's metabolism copes with decay.
As we come to diagnose a state of relative strength and the
symptoms of an impaired one, we face only more clearly the
paradoxes and tragic potentials of human life" [4]. Erikson
refers to that adult retardation as stagnation that results in
eventual despair.

By way of review, it may be helpful to explain how the
various theories of development affect one's professional
functioning. Erikson's theory of psychosocial stages and

Freud's theory of psychosexual phases are the most well-developed psychological developmental theories. Those theories evolved from older developmental theories.

DEVELOPMENTAL THEORIES

During the twentieth century three major theories have affected American psychology and perhaps the nursing profession as well. One of these theories was the *social learning theory* of John B. Watson. Watson strongly influenced both professionals and parents. He believed that learning occurred through objective learning processes. He wrote extensively about shaping behavior (e.g., by developing habits of regularity, dependability, independence, and self-reliance). Watson advocated the instillation of certain behaviors, as the following excerpt from his works shows:

> There is a sensible way of treating children. Treat them as though they were young adults. Let your behavior always be objective and kindly firm. Never hug and kiss them, never let them sit in your lap. If you must, kiss them once on the forehead when they say good night. Shake hands with them in the morning . . . Try it out. In a week's time you will find how easy it is to be perfectly objective with your child . . . . [15]

Although Watson has been ridiculed and criticized in recent years, he had great influence at a time when emotional expression and experiences were considered expressions of instincts that should be "taught out of the child." Watson's approaches and social learning theories have been significantly altered in recent years. The work of Miller, Dollard, and Rotter on the control of infant and child behavior is more sophisticated and is more widely accepted.

Another theory of development that has probably influenced nursing's approach to care is the *maturational theory* of Arnold Gesell, which was influential in the 1940s and 1950s. Gesell was concerned with methods of developmental diagnosis and analysis based on norms of behavioral development. He was concerned with individual differences, and he thought that age norms should be established for standards of development — but only for purposes of orientation and interpretation. But

Gesell did not acknowledge that each person is different, often much different, from every other person.

Gesell's writings were very influential until the late 1940s. Then Benjamin Spock's *Baby and Child Care,* first published in 1945, displaced Gesell's work.

Watson and Gesell contributed the idea that professionals should educate parents about child development. Gesell believed that literature about child development should be in the home, and he considered the home the "cultural workshop" where human relationships were formed.

Many of those ideas of chronological maturational norms, social conditioning, dissemination of information, and individual differences are still influential. The growth and development charts that are seen in doctors' offices and in clinics show the influence of the maturational theory. Also, there is some carry-over of Watson's views in that some parents think they must not be too affectionate and they must "train bad impulses out of the child." That view is in sharp contrast to Spock's warm, close, permissive environment. Spock advocates a love and acceptance between parent and child that encourages the development of the inherent good nature of the child.

Recent times have been perhaps most influenced by the theories of psychoanalysis. Freud, the first psychoanalyst, and the neo-Freudians explained and described many phases of development. Their explanations and descriptions guide nurses' interventions. More recently, Erikson has provided a framework for studying the development of a person from birth through old age from a psychosocial perspective. Classic Freudian theory is generally considered a biological theory. It holds that biological drives are manifested entirely in a social context. For example, the "oral period" of infancy is concerned with the basic drive (or instinct) for sucking and eating. It is gratified by early interactions with one's parents, primarily one's mother. The manner in which the mother, or mother figure, gives determines the gratification and successful resolution of the oral period. Erikson, on the other hand, although he also is analytical, extends the oral stage into the psychosocial conflict that is necessary for resolution; namely, learning *trust* through the oral process and feeding and learning hope through the environmental object relationships. Although Freud would talk about fixation at that or other periods if the basic instinct was not gratified, Erikson refers to the counter-balancing force that always operates for psychosocial maintenance. For example, he considers mistrust the counterbalance of trust. Without successful resolution the dynamic force pulls toward mistrust and that movement affects the next stage of development.

Erikson developed an epigenetic chart that represents the normal sequence of psychosocial gains (see figure). These psychosocial gains are consistent with Freud's psychosexual stages.

In his chart, Erikson assumes that:

1. The human personality (in principle) develops according to steps that are predetermined by the growing person's readiness to be driven toward, to be aware of, and to interact with a widening circle of people.
2. Society (in principle) meets and invites those steps toward interaction, and it safeguards and encourages the proper rate sequence of the unfolding of the steps [4].

Erikson's view is that psychosocial development proceeds by critical steps, with "critical step" referring to a potential turning point in a person's life toward progress and regression or toward integration and retardation. The *critical nature* of the stages, combined with the *environment,* can lead to successful development of potentialities, and help safeguard and encourage the person so that the steps proceed in the proper sequence and at the proper rate.

The knowledge and understanding of (1) the healthy psychosocial stages and unhealthy counterforces, (2) the critical nature of the stages as turning points, and (3) the environmental impact role are useful to nursing from a primary health standpoint. Furthermore, such knowledge and understanding is important for nursing study and research that will extend the knowledge base and contribute to the understanding of human development. Such continued study and research, based on

FREUD'S PSYCHOSEXUAL STAGES

	1	2	3	4	5	6	7	8
8. Old age								Ego integrity versus despair
7. Mature adulthood							Generativity versus stagnation	
6. Young adulthood						Intimacy versus isolation		
5. Puberty and adolescence					Identity versus role confusion			
4. Latency				Industry versus inferiority				
3. Locomotor-genital stage			Initiative versus guilt					
2. Muscular-anal stage		Autonomy versus shame and doubt						
1. Oral-sensory stage	Basic trust versus mistrust							

ERIKSON'S PSYCHOSOCIAL STAGES

Erikson's psychosocial developmental stages (corresponding to Freud's psychosexual stages). (Adapted from Erikson [4]) successful observation and practice, will further the scientific base of caring.

The epigenetic diagram on page 251 suggests areas in which more work and research are needed. The epigenetic diagram helps the reader to compare the works of Freud and Erikson. It explains the psychodynamic forces and counterforces that work in the developmental process throughout life (not just through adolescence, as Freud suggested). Erikson's stages from young adulthood through old age are new and important contributions to the view of psychosocial conflicts, crises, and turning points beyond the psychosexual infant-childhood developmental sequences.

NEGOTIATION-RENEGOTIATION OF CONFLICTS

The *negotiation-renegotiation* aspect of the early childhood forces and counterforces that are actively occurring through-out life has not been emphasized enough in nursing knowledge and practice. The following paragraphs describe how that aspect of psychosocial development can provide nursing with a more scientific understanding of the psychological and social dimensions of the delivery of health care, especially holistic health care.

During the trust-distrust oral stage of development, the infant learns to test his or her environment and, through expe-riencing feeding, handling, responsiveness, protection, and safety on a day-to-day basis, the infant *learns* about self, signifi-cant others, and the world. The world is either predictable or unpredictable, satisfying or frustrating, safe or unsafe, secure or insecure, warm or cold, loving or hostile. Through experi-encing and feeling, the child begins from birth to negotiate what life is in relation to self, others, and the environment. Through a series of mutual exchanges (givings and receivings), the child and the environment fit or attempt to fit each other. That is the beginning of the formation of the child's character and personality in terms of one's life in relation to others. Beginning with the establishment of trust in others and in the environment, which is counterbalanced by experiences that provoke mistrust, the child learns an interchange that, it is hoped, results in trust and hope. As the child continues to give and take with the environment, he or she tries to achieve a balance by negotiating and renegotiating his or her own behavior according to the responses of the environment.

Each developmental stage is affected by not only the maintenance of the previous resolution (e.g., trust-hope or continued resolution attempts if the first stage was inadequate) but also by new dimensions of environmental exchange (e.g., autonomy and self-control). With those new dimensions, the child obtains a separate but complementary fit with self, others, and the environment. So the new developmental needs create new conflicts and new counterforces that require new negotiations between self, one's own behavior, and others. Likewise, the previous conflicts may have to be renegotiated, as the following paragraphs show.

The infant struggles with trusting the environment and through daily experiences develops a sense of what to expect. The infant, from a very early age, has a blueprint of the expectations of others about himself or herself. As the infant moves into the second and third years of life, the original blueprint for trust-hope may no longer work because of many new events in the child's life; for example, the child may be separated from his or her mother and exposed to other caretakers at home or at nursery school. At that point, while the child is learning new ways to control his life — to develop autonomous behaviors of self in relation to others — he or she may need to renegotiate (psychodynamically within and psychosocially with the environment) his or her previous expectations for trust-hope. The problem is compounded by the counterforce of the particular developmental sequence.

The psychosocial blueprints for one's self in relation to environmental or other expectations need to be questioned, and renegotiated throughout one's life. It is in that psychodynamic, primitive sense that everyone is struggling through life with basic psychosocial issues in order to become a fully mature and healthy human being. It is in that sense that different stages of life are "critical" turning points (toward health or illness) that can be considered developmental crises because of the personal and social conflicts that each new stage introduces or reactivates.

As indicated earlier, self-actualization may be the hallmark of health. If nurses try to understand and resolve their own developmental conflicts through self-awareness and a knowledge of developmental psychology, they can better understand the negotiations and renegotiations of conflicts that people struggle with throughout life. They can better assess and appreciate the stress-related issues of change in living situations — change in family constellation, death, loss, retirement, marriage, birthing, parenting, and role change. By examining a change while considering perceived stress, nurses can understand how much a patient must cope because of the external forces of change and, perhaps more important, the internal forces and counterforces related to negotiating developmental conflicts. Change of any kind, good or bad, makes a person test or renegotiate basic issues, such as trust, safety, security, separateness, ownership, and control.

To illustrate — consider the case of a well-adjusted young woman who has experienced the personal trauma of rape. Even though the woman may have resolved the developmental conflicts that occur during young adulthood (e.g., trust-hope, autonomy—will-power, initiative-purpose, industry-competence, and identity-fidelity), the rape would have disrupted her psychosocial equilibrium and made her renegotiate many of her previous resolutions. The trauma of rape provides the counterforce of resolution by threatening the resolutions made in the past (i.e., the counterforce of trust, raising the questions, Where am I safe? Who can protect me? How competent am I to protect myself? Do I have no control?).

Such a process of regression-retardation occurs normally as a response to many stress-change events in daily life. Many common life events (in addition to the unusual types of stress-change, such as rape) require a renegotiation between self and environment in regard to developmental conflicts. All the normal changes and stresses are augmented by the forces and counterforces that occur within the normal developmental stages or sequences.

So far, the following basic facts about developmental conflicts have been discussed:

1. Everyone must cope with psychosocial developmental conflicts at particular developmental stages.
2. Everyone must renegotiate previous resolved or unresolved conflicts from earlier developmental stages.
3. Each developmental stage, and perhaps each stress-change situation in life, can be viewed as a critical psychosocial turning point toward health or illness.
4. Nursing intervention should consider stress-change and developmental stages, following a developmental conflict model for holistic health care.
5. Since nursing care assesses potentialities, strengths, and environmental and psychosocial variables, holistic health care delivery can become as systematic and scientific as traditional secondary health care.

The following paragraphs further illustrate the significance of developmental conflicts by discussing what I call latent issues or latent themes. The issues or themes are associated with the more commonly known stages of growth and development. Perhaps the discussion will illuminate the larger symbolic and psychodynamic issues that are related to each stage. When either the basic developmental conflicts identified by Erikson or the latent surrounding issues that I have identified are activated, a negotiating-renegotiating process may take place in the particular individual. Table 12-1 identifies the latent themes related to the major developmental stages. It may help to sort out and describe some of the complexities of the developmental conflict model.

As Table 12-1 shows, there are other latent issues and psychosocial processes that can accompany specific developmental conflicts. Table 12-1 provides another way to look at the complex psychosocial aspects of individual development. As Table 12-1 shows, basic safety and other expectations stem from very early experiences. When the basic issues are threatened later in life, (e.g., by illness, separation from parents, an unfamiliar environment), the early expectations and resolutions surrounding those basic issues undergo a retesting, reexamination, and renegotiation. The renegotiation, as well as the original negotiation of the basic psychosocial conflicts,

Table 12-1. Latent Psychosocial Processes Related to Erikson's Stages to Be Negotiated and Renegotiated Throughout Life

Erikson's Development Stages	Primary Processes (Positive Psychosocial Forces to Be Negotiated and Renegotiated)	Secondary Processes (Counter Psychosocial Forces That Need to Be Renegotiated)
Infant		
Stage 1:		
Basic trust	Safety	Lack of safety
versus	Security	Insecurity
distrust	Dependency	Independency
	Hope	Hopelessness
Toddler		
Stage 2:		
Autonomy	Internal self-control	External control
versus	Pride	Shame
shame and	Self-confidence	Self-criticism
doubt	Creativity-spontaneity	Inhibition
	Possession-ownership	Possession
	Giving	Retaining
	Freedom	Restriction
	Helpfulness	Helplessness
Preschooler		
Stage 3:		
Initiative	Independence-inter-	Dependence
versus	dependence	
guilt	Positive sexual	Negative view of own
	identity	sexuality
	("good me")	Negative self-image
		(bad me")
	Family-role identi-	Faulty family-role iden-
	fication	tification
	Positive self-image	Self-promise
	Self-acceptance	Self-punishment
	Positive orientation to	Negative orientation to
	authority (moral	authority
	development)	
School-age Child		
Stage 4:		
Industry	Self-assurance	Feeling of defeat
versus	Task mastery	Task failure
inferiority	Learning confidence	Learning insecurity

Table 12-1 (continued)

Erikson's Development Stages	Primary Processes (Positive Psychosocial Forces to Be Negotiated and Renegotiated)	Secondary Processes (Counter Psychosocial Forces That Need to Be Renegotiated)
	Cooperation	Difficulty with cooperative relationship
	Capability-competence	Lack of capability-incompetence
	Openness and problem-solving ability	Resistance to problem solving
Adolescent Stage 5: Identity versus role confusion	Internal stability Self-acceptance Heterosexual resolution Questioning authority	Internal instability Self-rejection Heterosexual conflict Submissive-rebellious to authority
Young Adult Stage 6: Intimacy versus isolation	Affiliation-love Relationship commitment Separateness from family	Loneliness Lack of commitment Dependency on family
Nurturing and Parenting/ Mature Adult Stage 7: Generativity versus stagnation	Productivity-achievement Caring, giving to others External challenges Contributions to society	Nonproductive-nonachieving Self-absorption Preoccupation with internal conflicts Fear of success
Old Age Stage 8: Ego integrity versus despair	Approval of self Self-satisfaction Psychosocial negotiations successful Contentment-wisdom	Self-recrimination Regrets Unresolved psychosocial negotiations Remorse-discontent

may be a critical turning point toward health or illness. Therefore people can be helped in health maintenance by the nurse
who understands the psychosocial aspects of developmental
conflicts.

Basic developmental conflicts, struggles, and latent psychosocial processes are ongoing. Many of the conflicts from birth
through adolescence become manifested again in different
degrees and different forms in the young-adult, mature-adult,
and old-age periods. Healthy coping depends on past resolutions, past and present environmental stresses, accuracy of perceptions, renegotiation attempts, and present supports.

PERCEPTIONS, COPING, AND NURSING
INTERVENTIONS

As Table 12-1 shows, a pattern of perceiving self and others
gradually develops and sets the stage for a pattern of coping
with internal and external stresses and conflicts.

Some of the coping patterns have been described in the
literature. They are related to stress transactions between a
developing person and his or her environment. Depending on
earlier negotiations between self and others, stress throughout
the life cycle can be perceived by the experiencing person as
harm, loss, threat, or challenge-growth [9].

The perceptions of harm, loss, and threat stem from a negative evaluation of one's present or future well-being. The
perception of challenge-growth provides the least negative
connotation and the most positive view of stress.

A *harm-loss* perception is related to development that has
already occurred. For example, (1) a change in one's self concept or body image has already occurred, (2) one has left the
family's household, or (3) one has experienced an interpersonal loss. The coping responses for resolving the stress of the
past may still operate. Unresolved feelings of harm-loss (real
or imaginary) can carry over into other transactions and result
in some form of illness.

Developmental threats can involve harm or loss that is anticipated but that has not yet happened, such as emancipation
from parents, loss of job, approach of retirement, fears about

the death of parents, one's spouse, or one's self. Developmental threats may also be associated with taking on new experiences, school work, intimate relationships, social-community activities, or financial responsibilities.

Developmental challenges are the most interesting view of developmental conflicts. An orientation toward challenge rather than threat or harm may be a most important force for motivating people to deal with their psychosocial development.

Nursing interventions during developmental conflict or stress may be directed to changing the perception of the developmental stress from that of threat to that of challenge and growth. The change in perception may alter the meaning of the stress, clarify any distortion of the stress, and promote health. Intervention directed toward changing a troubled transaction between perceptions and actions is referred to as *instrumental* intervention [9].

If the intervention is directed toward support and regulation of the emotions involved in the developmental conflict, it can be classified as an *expressive* intervention. Both kinds of nursing interventions are necessary and appropriate for different persons at different times. The choice of interventions depends on (1) the *perception* the person has of the developmental stress, (2) the *coping mechanisms* the person may use (e.g., information seeking, direct action, inhibition of actions, or intrapsychics [9], and (3) the *situational supports* (e.g., the support of family, friends, and colleagues).

Expressive interventions promote cognitive and affective coping and perhaps lead to more direct actions or information seeking and better utilization of the available situational supports.

Instrumental interventions impart cognitive information through teaching-learning and attempts to alter the meaning of the developmental stress, clarify distortions of threat, or alter the troubled transactions between the person and his or her environmental supports.

In general, coping is an interaction between the person and his or her environment. It consists of all the efforts made by a person to manage demands that tax or exceed his or her resources [9].

The following are specific ways of coping with developmental stress:

1. *Effective Action.* Action on self or the environment that has an external and interpersonal orientation. Effective action tries to repair damage or prevent future damage. It can include anticipatory coping to prepare for the stresses of the next developmental task. Anticipatory coping may reduce the threat of the next task and increase the challenge-growth value of the developmental tasks at hand. Effective coping also includes confronting chronic low-level threatening situations throughout life — the day-to-day pressures and hassles of living [9]. Often that kind of coping activity, while not dramatic, is most important to health and illness. Constant struggles and one's orientation and perception of them may reflect agendas from past experiences, a renegotiation of unresolved developmental conflicts. Intervention with action may be directed toward changing a person's perceptions, thinking, and previous modes of action that were not successful in managing the demands that tax the person's resources.

   Since the demands that tax or exceed a person's resources can be external or internal, internal-intrapsychic cognitive processes may also help the person cope effectively.

2. *Lowering of Stress Level.* Lowering of stress level can occur internally or cognitively; for example, by denial (which can be positive or negative) or by changing the significance and meaning of the stress.

   Some people are more responsive to planning-type and action-type coping responses, whereas others respond better to internal-intrapsychic, cognitive processes. There are also unknown mechanisms that help in coping. People protect themselves by a variety of mechanisms. It is not known what mechanism works; success usually depends on the circumstances and the people. But even though much is not known about coping, the two broad categories just discussed can help the nurse.

Knowing a person's method of coping helps determine before nursing interventions are planned, what a person does or does not do or what works. The nurse can begin to problem solve within a developmental stress context, deciding either to try to alter the person-environment situation, or not to try to change the situation but to plan interventions in order to lower the person's response to the stress.

The nurse can play a vital role in preventive health care by knowing and anticipating the developmental stresses that commonly occur during each life phase. In addition, the nurse can choose purposeful interventions after she or he assesses the person's perception of the developmental stress, the methods of coping that work or do not work, and the availability and kind of situational forces that influence the person.

There are two types of nursing interventions:

1. *Interventions That Attempt to Change the Perceptions and Thus Lower the Stress* [9]. Such interventions are primarily cognitive, teaching-learning strategies combined with the expressive interventions of counseling and emotional support. The goal would be lowering of the stress level and support of the internal-intrapsychic resources to help a person cope effectively.
2. *Interventions That Attempt to Change the Behaviors of the Person-Environment Transactions*. Such interventions encourage effective action because of their external-interpersonal focus. The goal would be to help the person repair the damage or to prevent future damage. The patient may prevent damage by anticipatory coping. In anticipatory coping, the patient reduced the threat of a situation by preparing himself or herself for it. The mother and child who have been gradually and occasionally separated before the child begins school have engaged in anticipatory coping.

The nurse who understands that each phase of human growth brings conflicts that affect present and future development and health gives more serious attention to the importance of coping assessments and planned nursing interventions that promote health throughout the life span — and before a person becomes a "patient." Often there is a long period of time between the perception of developmental stress and exhausting one's coping and becoming ill. Nursing interventions that key coping management of developmental stress to specific early responses of the person can promote primary prevention at a high level of effectiveness.

FAMILY DEVELOPMENTAL CONFLICTS

The evidence suggests that the family as well as the individual has sequential stages of growth and development and therefore developmental conflicts. The following discussion outlines some of the characteristics of family development that the student and practicing nurse might meet in working with families.

If one assumes that a young adult couple has resolved the intimacy-versus-isolation conflict by falling in love and deciding to marry and have a family, one can also assume that the couple has entered a family developmental cycle. The cycle discussed in the following paragraphs is a normal one, and it has many variations. Variations are common today because of the great variety of life-styles of young adults, as shown by the increase in the number of single-parent families, divorces, remarriages, adoptions, and so on.

Nevertheless, it is helpful to view the sequential stages of family life (1) as a basis of comparison with individual development and (2) as a basis for identifying critical turning points for family growth and development in order to plan nursing intervention in health maintenance and prevention of illness.

The stages of the family's developmental cycle have been identified as [2, 8] :

1. The establishment stage
2. The new-parent stage
3. The pre-school-age-children stage
4. The school-age-children stage
5. The adolescent-children stage
6. The launching-center stage

7. The post-parental stage
8. The aging-family stage

The labeling is consistent with the social and chronological movement of children into and through the family and out into society, with a post-parental stage in which the children have left home and the parents grow old.

From a psychosocial standpoint, each of these family stages could upset an established pattern or equilibrium and create a situation of stress, harm, loss, threat, or challenge. Each stage may be a developmental conflict one that may require renegotiation of basic psychosocial issues related to individual development. The family developmental conflict can also be aggravated by the basic developmental conflict related to the current stage of individual development.

The *establishment* phase begins with marriage, and it is characterized by the couple's functioning as a dyad. The phase continues until the first child is born. Preparation for the birthing and parenting experiences is a neglected area of health care. Even the anticipation of change in the dyad is stressful enough to create a critical turning point. If that stress is aggravated by conflicts regarding intimacy and isolation, health maintenance is understandably difficult.

The *new-parent* stage begins with pregnancy and the birth of the first child. The shift in roles from wife to wife and mother and husband to husband and father is a major change that requires coping. To become totally responsible for another person is a demanding, stressful experience. Research findings [10] report that a high percentage of families studied (83 percent) had a "severe" or "extensive" crisis with the birth of the first child. The conclusion of the study was that the crisis occurred not because the child was unwanted or the marriage was unhappy or the couple was maladjusted, but because the couples had little or no preparation for parenthood. The conclusion has important intervention implications for nursing in the delivery of health care. It indicates that parenthood can be a turning point toward health or illness for parents and for the infant, thus setting up another cycle of developmental conflicts.

The following paragraphs discuss the recent findings regarding bonding between the parents (especially the mother) and the infant. In health care delivery/settings, health professionals, and nurses in particular, have become aware of the advantages of preparing for the birthing experience as well as for parenting.

Natural childbirth, or an approach similar to natural childbirth, is strongly advocated. With natural childbirth, the mother can be alert during the birth because she has been given a minimum of anesthetics and analgesics. Furthermore, she has practiced breathing, relaxation, and exercises long before her baby is born. If the husband takes part — as he often does — the birthing experience can be an even more successful and satisfying one.

During labor, the mother-to-be participates to the fullest degree possible. At the delivery, she is awake and alert, and she immediately holds and cuddles her baby. It is believed that the contact immediately (within minutes) after delivery is critical to the development of a bond between the mother and baby that contributes to a more intimate, loving, and protective relationship between them. Some researchers believe that the bonding is a type of imprinting that sets the foundation for the first developmental stage — the development of trust. Some researchers think that without bonding, the development of trust may be impeded. Some also think that bonding may decrease the child-battering potentials of parents.

A specific systematic process is believed to occur that is related to the mother's looking at and then touching the newborn baby, first with her fingers, then with her entire hand until the baby's whole body is embraced by the mother. Because the mother has been given a minimum amount of anesthetics, the infant, also is alert and responsive, and he or she looks at, smells, and feels the mother. It is believed that through the bonding process, security and trust are established at that moment. The bond can also include the father. Nursing knowledge and interventions related to prepared childbirth and to bonding are important primary preventive activities. A satisfying birthing experience and the establishment of a bond between the infant and parent are now considered essential for the health of both.

The *pre-school-age-children* stage of family development is another critical family stage. In that stage, the oldest child is between three and six years old. The tasks for the family include nurturing, child-rearing, and managing the financial resources for the bigger family. At the same time the couple tries to maintain intimacy in the relationship. Some researchers have suggested that as the child grows and progresses through the psychosexual and psychosocial stages of development, the parents' previous developmental conflicts are reactivated and have to be renegotiated.

The *school-age-children* stage brings stress and change when the oldest child enters school full time. Often the mother may return to work at that point, creating another change. Preparations for the parents' need and opportunities for growth are important intervention issues for health at that critical turning point. Parents, especially the mother, experience a real and symbolic loss when the child leaves the home. Even with preparation, the event can still be difficult for the family, and it can affect the developing child also.

The *adolescent-children* stage begins when the oldest child reaches puberty. The developmental tasks for the family include a growth in the child's independence, mobility, sexuality, beginning of mate selection, beginning thoughts of a career choice, and selection of a college. Authority control, renegotiating previous developmental tasks, and conflicts because of alcohol and drugs are common at that stage.

Communication and closeness are important for parents and adolescents, although the authority-dependency conflict sometimes supersedes and interferes with the family communication. Families can often benefit from communication or counseling concerning those issues.

The *launching-center* stage occurs when the oldest child departs from the family — for college, separate living quarters, marriage, and so on. At that time parents undergo stress because of the changes related to giving up the child and trusting the past developmental strengths and resolutions to help the child mature on his or her own. Again, the turning point may cause the parents to reactivate old conflicts about their growth, maturity and separateness from their own parents — conflicts that may have to be renegotiated when their son or daughter leaves. The launching stage is further complicated by the occurrence of menopause. When the child leaves, the mother experiences the "empty nest" syndrome, making the stage a potentially critical one because of the stress-change, loss, and developmental conflicts that occur simultaneously.

The *post-parental* stage occurs after the youngest child has left the home for his or her own career, separate living quarters, marriage, and so on. The stage is usually marked by independence, freedom and high earnings for the parents. The time coincides with the generativity period in the parents' individual development. However, it can be a critical turning point because of the difficulties connected with the loss. The post-parental stage often coincides with the need to care for elderly parents, grieving over the loss of one's parents, changing roles by becoming grandparents, and anticipating one's own old age. The grandparent role can be a source of great satisfaction and fulfillment during the post-parental stage.

The *aging-family* stage is characterized by the retirement of the husband and often the wife too. The severe losses in role, self-concept, self-image, routine, and personal relationships are complicated by a decline in finances. If the couple can adjust successfully, they can enjoy much satisfaction and pleasure through children and grandchildren, their freedom to travel and to engage in postponed activities and civic events, and so on. Some elderly persons and couples even return to college to work on a degree or take courses that they are interested in. Anticipation of one's own death and the death of one's spouse is also a concern during the aging-family stage. The concern about death should not be ignored; it could lead to a sense of closure of and satisfaction with one's life, as well as to a sense of integrity.

SUMMARY
The eight stages of the family developmental cycle have been discussed as part of developmental conflicts. The fact that family development is an important issue and a focus for concern makes it an important area for nursing to study. Comparing

the individual developmental stages with the family developmental stages is also useful. Knowledge of psychosocial conflicts that affect health is essential to health care delivery, because the conflicts that occur during the various stages can be critical turning points toward health or illness. Health preparation and interventions related to the stages and conflicts may help individual families to cope better. Health maintenance and illness prevention result from primary and holistic health care intervention related to individual and family developmental conflicts.

Chapter 13 discusses loss, a human condition and normal life process that is important for health and the science of care.

REFERENCES

1. Benedek, T. *Psychosexual Functions in Women.* New York: Ronald, 1952.
2. Duvall, E. M. *Family Development* (4th ed.). Philadelphia: Lippincott, 1971.
3. Engel, G. *Psychological Development in Health and Disease.* Philadelphia: Saunders, 1963.
4. Erikson, E. H. *Childhood and Society* (2nd ed.). New York: Norton, 1963.
5. Gesell, A. *Youth: The Years from Ten to Sixteen.* New York: Harper & Bros., 1956.
6. Gesell, A., and Ilg, F. L. *Infant and Child in the Culture of Today.* New York: Harper & Bros., 1943.
7. Hill, R. *Family Development in Three Generations.* Cambridge, Mass.: Schenkman, 1971.
8. Kimmel, D. *Adulthood and Aging.* New York: Wiley, 1974.
9. Lazarus, R. S., and Launier, R. Stress-related Transactions Between Person and Environment. In L. A. Pervin and M. Lewis (eds.), *Interaction Between Internal and External Determinants of Behavior.* New York: Plenum, 1978.
10. LeMasters, E. E. Parenthood as crisis. *Marriage and Family Living* 19:453, 1957.
11. Liebert, T. M., Poulos, R. W., and Strauss, G. D. *Developmental Psychology.* Englewood Cliffs, N.J.: Prentice-Hall, 1974.
12. Miller, N. E., and Dollard, J. *Social Learning and Imitation.* New Haven, Conn.: Yale University Press, 1953.
13. Murray, R., and Zentner, J. *Nursing Assessment and Health Promotion Through the Life Span.* Englewood Cliffs, N.J.: Prentice-Hall, 1975.

14. Rotter, J. B. *Social Learning and Clinical Psychology.* Englewood Cliffs, N.J.: Prentice-Hall, 1954.
15. Rotter, J. B., Chance, J. E., and Phares, E. J. *Application of a Social Learning Theory of Personality.* New York: Holt, Rinehart and Winston, 1972.
16. Watson, J. B. *Psychological Care of Infant and Child.* London: Allen & Unwin, 1928.

13. LOSS

Loss as a concept and as an experience is present throughout life. Most people, however, think of loss only in terms of obvious, tangible, concrete losses, such as the loss of a significant person through death, the loss of a home through disaster, or the loss of smaller possessions (e.g., a piece of jewelry, purse, wallet, or coat). In reality, however, loss is a highly variable personal experience. What is loss to one person is not necessarily loss to another. Accordingly, loss can be understood only in terms of the meaning it has to the person involved in it.

Loss in its broadest sense exists when any aspect of one's self (whether tangible-concrete, intangible-abstract, real or imaginary) is no longer available to a person. Loss also exists when a valued object (including a person) is altered for an individual. The following Greek proverb captures the idea of loss as a symbolic yet real experience throughout life — "One experiences loss of childhood at 12, loss of youth at 18, loss of love at 20, loss of faith at 30, loss of hope at 40, and loss of desire at 50" [1]. Such a cynical view of life may not be healthy, but the proverb makes it clear that loss is not only tangible, concrete, and physical but also symbolic and personal, that loss can be fully known only by the person experiencing it.

Loss can refer to loss of the image one has of one's self and one's body — one's private and social identity. Loss can be associated with loss of one's body image and physique and one's self-representation. With that association come symbolic, abstract, psychological, and sociocultural meanings connected to self-identity, self-concept, one's ideas and feelings about one's self, worth, beauty, desirability, capabilities, and other special qualities. All these factors contribute to the meaning that loss has for the person who for some reason is deprived of certain characteristics.

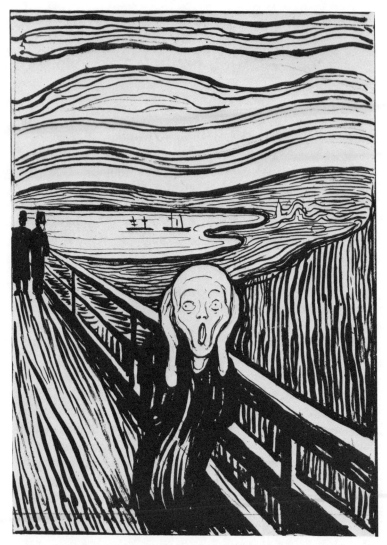

Geschrei, by Edward Munch. (Collection, Oslo Kommunes Kunstsamlinger, Munch-Museet)

The loss experience depends on the perspective, values, and meanings that the loss has for the person experiencing it.

In a general sense then, loss can be conceptualized in (1) *psychological terms* (e.g., loss of self-concept, self-esteem, or self-identity), (2) *sociocultural terms* (e.g., loss of social identity, social role, family constellation, or cultural heritage), and (3) *physical terms* (e.g., loss of body function or structure or loss in quality of valued physical attributes).

All types of loss occur as normal and vital parts of life. Loss affects everyone from birth until death. Some losses are haphazard and unpredictable, others are overt and tangible, and still others may be sudden or gradual, and tangible or abstract and symbolic. Certain losses are necessary for growth and development throughout life.

Loss is an inherent component of all changes in life, both positive and negative ones. Even though positive changes are not normally viewed as loss, theorists and researchers of loss indicate that even changes that bring gain (as in marriage and job promotion) also bring an experience of loss. The loss may be primarily psychological, sociocultural, or physical — or it may be a combination of all those factors.

Regardless of its origin, nature, or meaning, loss affects everyone's adjustment, coping, and adaptation throughout life. A loss can be a crucial one that requires preparation, anticipation, and planned interventions for its successful resolution. The science of caring needs to understand loss in a comprehensive sense in order to deliver primary health care. Loss is differentiated for comprehensive learning purposes into psychological loss, sociocultural loss, and physical loss.

PSYCHOLOGICAL LOSS
Psychological loss is an unconscious or subconscious phenomenon. Development of the psychological self is a gradual process of self-awareness that begins at birth. It includes visual, tactile, structural, and postural perceptions, as well as cognitive and affective states associated with one's total functioning self. Throughout the periods of growth and development, people gain energy from attaching themselves to

significant persons and objects. Those significant others become incorporated into the self in a total developing sense.
The incorporation includes the symbolism and meanings
attached to the others, which become part of the psychological self. One's concept of his or her psychological self forms
a nucleus for one's personality and coping. As one continues
to grow physically and mentally, certain psychological changes
occur. The affective states associated with total self and the
inherent changes determine the meaning, values, and intensity
of the loss of the psychological self.

The figure on page 273 shows the inherent growth and developmental loss experiences associated with living. From
birth until death, each person moves through life and its inherent processes in a unique way. Different experiences from
birth to death are critical issues at different points in life. All
life changes are in some way experiences of loss, and they
require coping and readjustment. The life line represents a
person's movement through life, with different developmental
issues being critical at certain points. The issues present themselves in unique and varying patterns and thereby affect the
meaning of loss for the particular person.

The psychological forms of loss involve the affective, cognitive, and symbolic aspects of self as well as the developmental
loss that is a necessary concomitant of growth and development. As one matures, one experiences a great number of
losses (e.g., of the pleasures associated with security, comfort,
dependency, and protectedness). Even though the developmental changes associated with "growing up" are positive and
provide new gains for a person, they include frustrating and
tangible and intangible losses. The experience of those losses
is altered by the quality, quantity, and intensity of the loss, as
well as by the perceived meaning of the loss. Such psychological and developmental losses can create a negative and
lifelong impression on the developing personality. There is
increasing evidence that the personality continues to develop
throughout life and that symbolic and real losses continue.

Each loss is a reality that has personal and symbolic meanings for the person experiencing it. What one person perceives
as a gain another may perceive as a loss. Symbolic psychological

Developmental Loss Factors	Conception	Critical Periods
Loss of symbiosis		Birth/infancy
Loss of total dependency		Toddlerhood
Loss of parental attachment		Preschool stage
Loss of family circle as primary unit		School-age stage
Loss of childhood securities; loss of self-image		Adolescence
Loss of role in family		Young adulthood
Loss of youth/freedom		Adulthood
Loss of children; some loss of physical processes		Middle adulthood
Loss of established roles and relationships; often loss of health		Old age
Loss of life	Death	

Loss experiences inherent in human development throughout life.

losses or even anticipated losses may produce intense, stressful responses that are unique to each person and that are related to existing coping-adaptive mechanisms.

Each loss contains the threat of an additional loss. Each loss is affected by the quality, quantity, and intensity of one's previous losses and one's success in coping with them. For example, in old age the loss of certain behaviors (e.g., the loss of independence) also involves the loss of one's role and of certain self-images and the loss of the acceptance by others of one's former self. The resolution (or lack of resolution) of the loss determines the perception of the next loss experience.

Different developmental stages are vulnerable times for certain symbolic loss — psychologically and developmentally: infancy, toddlerhood, preschool period, school-age period, latent period, adolescence, young adulthood, middle adulthood, older adulthood, and old age. The defensive and adaptive skills for handling loss are relatively few until adolescence, when they increase, reaching maximum development in the adult years and then diminishing in old age.

Even though loss occurs in all stages of life, infancy, childhood, adolescence, and old age are particularly vulnerable times for losses. However, in light of the new awareness of growth and development at all ages, it is becoming evident that the transition into so-called adulthood or maturity is a particularly crucial milestone of loss. The current young adult behaviors reflect a last struggle to "give up" the dependency, the protectedness, the opportunity to be guided by external figures in career and marital choices. Only when a person breaks into adulthood does he or she realize the struggle with loss that is part of becoming psychologically as well as physically mature. During the break into "maturity" one becomes completely responsible for self. During the adult years one experiences a deepening of values and an extension of interests and caring beyond the self.

Adjustment to a psychological loss, whether it is related to one's cultural heritage, social role, or self-image, can be as difficult as adjustment to loss of a body part. The process of coping is the same, involving an adaptation to a significant loss. The resolution of all losses requires coping and adaptation.

The losses of middle age include an altered body image and self-image. Although Jung, Erikson, and Sheehy consider middle age a time of positive gain (in regard to accomplishments, contributions, productivity, generativity, and "approval of oneself at last"), loss of the psychological self accompanies the growth and development of middle age and old age.

The aging process involves inherent developmental losses that accumulate and become greater with age. Even though

the "middle-aged–older-aged adult" is in the mainstream of
life, psychology has done little to help in the understanding of
the personality development that occurs in middle age. Yet
that is the time when one often feels "loss of hope" and "loss
of desire," the time when one is "over the hill" in the view of
young adults, the time of the "deadline decade . . . the time of
change in time sense, a time of groping toward authenticity,
a time for letting go of the impossible dream" [19].

The psychological loss experienced during old age can often
be the most depressing loss of all. One may experience not
only the normal psychological and biophysical changes, which
are losses, but also social, economic, and cultural changes.
Each aspect of loss can affect another aspect. The aged person
often experiences a profound sociocultural loss along with
psychological and biophysical loss. The loss may consist of a
significant role change – from (1) that of parent to that of
grandparent, (2) that of spouse to that of widow or widower,
(3) that of a friend of many to that of a friend of few (or
friendless), (4) that of an active participant in life to that of a
passive recipient of life, (5) that of the head of the family constellation to a position "outside" the family constellation,
(6) that of a member of a diverse culture to that of a member
of an aged culture (or subculture), (7) that of an economically
comfortable person to that of an economically threatened
person, or (8) a position of high status and power to a position
of low status and powerlessness.

Although developmental losses are constant and present in
varying degrees at all ages and positions in the life cycle, they
are often present in their most crystallized forms for the aged
person.

Summary
Psychological loss includes the whole range of attitudes toward
the self and emotional states as well as the views and feelings
associated with the constantly occurring changes.

The concept of psychological loss is abstract and symbolic;
it is different for each person. Psychological loss associated
with the inherent changes in self is personal. The concept of
psychological loss provides a dynamic orientation to the

understanding of loss. It includes overt loss as well as covert, symbolic loss; it accommodates real, imaginary, or perceived loss that stems from intrapsychic, interpersonal, or developmental processes. To appreciate psychological loss, one can examine some of his or her own life experiences and struggles to "grow up."

SOCIOCULTURAL LOSS

The concept of sociocultural loss is not a well-developed one, but such loss occurs as frequently as psychological loss. In fact, both types of loss often accompany and aggravate each other. The acculturation process that implodes in every person in U.S. society is a threat to one's sociocultural being.

The emphasis on material goods, consumption, and "bigger-is-better" still prevails in the United States, even though that orientation is gradually changing because of ecological concerns. The great social pressure to give up one's cultural heritage interferes with the individual's rights and desire to follow his or her cultural heritage and belief system.

Society's ideal of conformity places great pressure on those who are different in regard to values and beliefs. Pressure to conform often separates people from themselves and others. The changes in systems of behavior, role, life-style, and belief often contribute to the loss of sociocultural self. Such a loss is perhaps most obvious in U.S. society, in which people dream of "the good life," typified by the life of a white, middle-class family that has a big house, a big car, and money with which to buy more and more things. The pressure forces all people, regardless of their own values, belief systems, and past experiences, to become acculturated to the "American way of life."

A dramatic illustration of that pressure is the sociocultural loss experienced by the Vietnamese refugees. Their great loss of sociocultural identity began with the rapid evacuation of Vietnam over a three-week period in April and May, 1975 (after the resignation of the president of Vietnam and the collapse of the Saigon government) [20].

One-hundred-and-thirty-five thousand Vietnamese refugees came to the continental United States. To help them adjust, the Department of Health, Education, and Welfare conducted initial screening and cultural orientation and provided language programs. The refugees were also instructed in the "American way of life."

It is difficult to evaluate the benefits and hazards of such programs. The programs to acculturate the refugees have helped them to understand where they were and how U.S. society differed from their society, but the programs may also have brought about a more pronounced sense of loss of their own culture. Such a programmed transition from one culture to another may intensify an already felt psychological loss as well as tangible, object-environmental losses.

The Vietnamese refugees experienced a severe culture shock in its basic form. Culture shock (and, in the case of the Vietnamese, sociocultural loss) occurs when a person is

suddenly thrust into an alien culture or has divided loyalties to two different cultures. In its most extreme form it means facing new mores and values and unlearning all of the old automatic daily cues of social behavior [8].

The sociocultural losses experienced by the Vietnamese refugees included loss of country, language, employment, familiar food, family structure, religion, social structure, customs and life-style, and separation from family [13]. The reactions to such profound sociocultural losses were anger, remorsefulness, resentfulness, sadness, depression, and even psychotic breaks and suicide [2]. The help given the refugees often took the form of helping with the acculturation process rather than helping them to cope with their severe losses.

Resocializing, rehousing, and readjusting to a new culture and life-style can be a shattering experience that involves profound loss. Family connections and past behaviors are often no longer condoned or even available. In many cultures domestic life and trade are often mingled, with a compactness of family and job networks that cannot be duplicated in a suburban American setting.

The reactions of families who were moved during an urban renewal project have been studied. Freud [10] and Marris [15] give examples of how sociocultural changes bring a sense of loss. Marris in particular warns social planners about the difficulties of change. A person who had been moved in a rehousing project in Boston's West End said that he felt that he "had lost everything" [15].

Marris described four kinds of sociocultural loss:

1. Loss of attachments
2. Disintegration of a predictable environment
3. Prospective threat to the meaning of life
4. Alteration of a relationship

Closely related to Marris's premise are the categories Glaser and Strauss [11] established for the different kinds of loss. Although Glaser and Strauss are referring to the kinds of losses that a dying person experiences, their categories can be applied to sociocultural loss.

1. Personal loss. Loss of attachments and involvements with others (similar to what Marris calls loss of attachments). Personal loss is related to the loss of psychological self.
2. Work loss. Loss of the meaning and significance of one's work (similar to what Marris calls prospective threat to the meaning of life and the disintegration of a predictable environment).
3. Social loss. Loss of events, objects, and people (similar to what Marris calls disintegration of a predictable environment, including family beliefs, the role of relatives, and religious, cultural, and day-to-day patterns of living).

Incorporating the concept of sociocultural loss into the concepts of psychological and biophysical loss permits a better understanding of overt and symbolic loss. Any change in the normal patterns of one's life or any disruption in one's daily routines and responsibilities is a loss. Such a view of loss includes the cognitive, affective, and behavioral losses that may operate within an individual. A comprehensive orientation to loss includes interpersonal, environmental, and intrapsychic processes.

Psychological and sociocultural losses may take many

different forms and meanings, depending on (1) the individual, (2) the extent of loss or change, (3) the extent to which the object lost was valued, (4) the manner in which the object lost was valued, (5) the number of previous losses, and (6) whether adequate coping and resolution occurred.

PHYSICAL LOSS

Physical loss is perhaps the most obvious and easily understood kind of loss. It involves external objects and possessions (such as the loss of home, money, or jewelry) or biophysical aspects of the body (such as loss of the body's function, structure, or appearance). In a sense, the concept of physical loss can be extended to include the loss of a loved or valued person through death, divorce, or separation. In a close, interdependent relationship, the loss of a significant other means the loss of certain aspects of one's physical self (as well as one's psychological and sociocultural selves). The physical self may be affected or incapacitated because of other types of loss of self (e.g., psychological loss and sociocultural loss). In such an instance of loss of a significant other, all kinds of loss operate at intense levels. According to Holmes, Rahe, and their co-workers, "loss of significant other" (e.g., by the death of a spouse) was found to create the highest amount of stress-crisis for people [12].

Even though physical loss includes loss of possessions and loss of significant others, the following discussion concentrates on the loss of one's immediate, tangible, physical self.

The loss of body function includes forms of loss of health. It is often seen as a change in one's self. It may even include such losses as loss of positive feelings about one's health and loss of contentment. Temporary, progressive, or permanent illnesses usually mean loss of body function. They may cause weakness, inactivity, pain, and fatigue or partial or total loss of a body function (such as breathing, bowel function, circulation, digestion, activity, sexual relations, vision, hearing, memory, cognition, and affective states).

Loss of body structure refers to the external, objective physical self. Loss of a tangible body part by trauma, amputation, surgery, or disease is considered a loss of body structure. Loss of body structure also includes loss of physical appearance and attractiveness and changes in the quality of the body's structure. Loss of body structure can refer to loss of internal or external body structures (e.g., loss of the uterus in a hysterectomy and loss of a breast in a mastectomy). It can also refer to the loss of physical beauty and other changes associated with age or illness.

Researchers and other workers who study loss have found that the symptoms of illness may remain even after medical intervention has eliminated the cause of the symptoms. The symptoms remain because they were incorporated into the person's self as a habitual part of the body's function or structure. The degree to which the symptoms were valued or provided secondary gain determines the person's capacity to "lose" them.

Each physical loss can threaten the person with an additional loss. For example, the loss of one's physical self may lead to the loss of one's psychological self-concept and the loss of one's role as an active participant with an established position in one's sociocultural environment.

The changes in one's physical self that are associated with the developmental stages, especially adolescence and old age, also result in a significant loss of one's physical self. The loss is accompanied by strong psychological and sociocultural factors that act concurrently.

The changes in physical functions, structures, and qualities that accompany old age are severe losses in U.S. culture, which has little regard for the aging body.

The loss associated with normal growth and development is continuous. In addition to the obvious loss of one's physical self that may occur with illness, surgery, or immobility, there is also the loss of one's physical self that occurs with aging.

When tangible physical loss occurs (such as loss from surgery), the evidence suggests that great psychological and sociocultural losses also occur. For example, an amputation can drastically injure one's self-concept (loss of one's psychological self). Likewise, the inability to engage in former roles or activities (e.g., as a breadwinner or as an athlete) extends the loss of one's physical self to a loss of one's sociocultural self.

Each loss carries with it other losses. All losses interact symbolically, and they are different for different people. The loss may be usual or unusual, real or imaginary. Regardless of whether the loss is physical, psychological or sociocultural, successful resolution requires the adaptive responses that affect all aspects of the self.

THE SYMBOLIC NATURE OF LOSS

Because of the dynamic and unique characteristics of each person, the meaning and significance of loss vary from person to person. In a recent clinical situation in which students were studying loss, a patient who had had both legs amputated was being interviewed. Even though the loss of his legs seemed to be the obvious and central loss, as the interview proceeded it became evident that the loss of his physical self was less significant to the man than a sociocultural loss he had experienced — the loss of his wife and children through a marital separation that had occurred several years before the amputation. Whenever loss was discussed with him, he talked about the amputation readily, realistically, and with optimism. But as the conversation continued, a *deeper* sense of loss emerged, a profound sociocultural loss. He was distressed that he was now all alone, living in a veterans' hospital, and alienated from his former sociocultural, physical self and from his role as husband and father.

Many variables affect loss. It is impossible to distinguish one part of loss; they all interact. Each loss carries with it other losses. And what seems to the viewer an obvious loss may be a different loss in the subjective, phenomenological view of the person experiencing the loss. Past meanings, associations, experiences, adjustments, and values establish a symbolic interaction that affects loss.

Loss is a universal and integral part of human experience that greatly affects everyone from birth to death. Some aspects of loss predictably accompany growth and development, whereas others are haphazard and unpredictable. Loss may take many different forms and have different meanings. Loss can be fully understood from the life space of the person who experiences it.

The nurse as a caring person needs to appreciate and value the symbolic and dynamic qualities of loss, which can be defined and interpreted more accurately and reliably by the person experiencing the loss.

The first part of this chapter discussed the concept of loss and the various components of loss — the psychological, sociocultural and physical components and their symbolic interactions. The rest of the chapter discusses some of the universal adaptive responses to loss that guide nursing intervention.

ADAPTATION TO LOSS

Grief and mourning are human behaviors that accompany loss. The terms grieving, mourning, bereavement, and grief work are used synonymously to refer to the processes that follow a loss and that help the mourner give up the lost object. Marris [15] indicated that grief work represents a struggle to retrieve a sense of meaning when meaning has been taken away by a loss.

Freud [9] defined mourning as a reaction to the loss of a loved person, object, or abstraction. He explained the grieving process as a phenomenon related to one's capacity for love (one's libido). Throughout growth and development, one's libido is diverted from one's own ego onto objects that are incorporated into one's ego. Loss of self includes not only loss of one's physical self but also the meanings of objects associated with one's self that have become incorporated into one's ego.

Detachment of the libido from one's self or from ego objects is a painful one. Freud said that the libido, for some unknown reason, clings to its objects and will not give them up when they are lost, even when substitutes are readily available.

Grief has been defined as a "universal subjective response following actual or anticipated loss of a valued object" [5]. Engel likened loss to a wound and mourning to the wound-healing process. Like wound healing, successful mourning involves an orderly sequence of events and an irreducible interval of time.

Various writers have described the characteristic phases of grieving. Engel [4] has identified the phases as:

1. The phase of shock and disbelief or denial
2. The phase of developing awareness of loss, which is accompanied by sadness, pain, helplessness, hopelessness, and crying
3. The phase of restitution, engaging in the rituals and intrapsychic work of dealing with the painful void

Lindemann [14] in his classic work on grief described the striking features of normal grief responses as:

1. Somatic distress, expecially of the digestive and respiratory systems
2. Preoccupation with the image of the lost object
3. Guilt
4. Hostility
5. Loss of one's normal behavior patterns (restlessness)

Parkes [16] identified the phases of grieving as similar to those in a stress-reaction: (1) alarm-restlessness, (2) fear, (3) searching for the lost object, (4) mitigation (i.e., feeling that the lost object is present), (5) guilt (alternating with depression, withdrawal, or apathy), and (6) new identity (incorporation of certain aspects of the loss into one's own behavior).

Anticipatory grief is another important aspect of grieving. In almost all the works on grief, anticipatory grief is described as any grief or grief work occurring before a loss, as distinguished from the grief that occurs *at* or *after* a loss.

A number of studies support the theory that anticipation may give a mourner a chance to carry out grief work before a loss. Expressing the pain and anguish of grief has been found to be appropriate, and it should be encouraged by nurses and other helping professionals.

Grief behaviors have been found to exist at any point in

grieving — from awareness to resolution. The consistent responses to loss reported in the works on grief are:

Helplessness	Depression
Loneliness	Withdrawal from people,
Sadness	events, and activities
Guilt	Extreme irritability
Self-deterioration	Restlessness
Anger	Preoccupation with the lost
Crying	object
Somatic distress (especially	Inability to initiate meaning-
loss of appetite)	ful activity
sleeplessness	

In summary, loss is related to higher order concepts of health in that quality of living is dependent to some degree on coping with normal changes and loss throughout all stages of growth and development. Furthermore, self-awareness, self-understanding, and acceptance of the loss may contribute to stress reduction and to a better resolution of the loss, resulting in a higher quality of living.

Recent research evidence suggests that loss associated with life changes (psychological, sociocultural, or physical changes) may play a significant role in the development of various physical and psychological (and perhaps even social) disorders [12].

Even though loss varies from one person to another, there is a consistency in the grief responses. Loss is a symbolic abstract process that is unique to the life space of the person experiencing it. In this sense, loss and its effects can be understood from a psychodynamic orientation rather than from a tangible, obvious interpretation. As professionals working with individuals, families, and groups of all ages, nurses must recognize the universal, symbolic nature of loss as a normal process from birth to death. Likewise, the nurse can anticipate, predict, and prepare people in regard to the grief behaviors that are necessary for further growth and resolution of loss.

Regardless of the nature of loss — whether it is normal, predictable, unexpected, or haphazard — the helping professional must (1) respond to the nature of the loss and the meaning it has for the person experiencing it and (2) facilitate the grief work that accompanies loss as a universal phenomenon of human behavior. Without proper grieving, the loss is not resolved. If the loss is not resolved, a person cannot cope with any future loss. The health professional who is familiar with the concept of loss and its many meanings and manifestations can promote coping and(or) grief work.

A health professional who understands the problems faced by the patient is truly responsive to health issues and can best raise the quality of the patient's life. Such a professional can give holistic health care that is primary, not secondary.

MANIFESTATIONS OF GRIEF AND RELATED NURSING INTERVENTIONS

The common manifestations of grief can be broken down into the following behaviors:

1. Denial (shock)
2. Anger (awareness)
3. Depression (relinquishment)
4. Reinvestment (resolution)

Table 13-1 gives examples of each of these behavioral manifestations of grief and of nursing interventions that are recommended for each one.

SUMMARY

Nursing can most effectively intervene in the common stressful processes of life, such as change, developmental conflict, and loss. Nursing, the science of caring, includes both humanistic and scientific approaches that help it respond to the need for holistic health care. Furthermore, the science of caring structures and orders study, practice, and research of the carative factors. Part III of this book has identified the concepts of holistic care and health that are relevant to consumer demands. Next, it identified the three major areas in which primary health interventions can help patients cope with

Table 13-1. Behavioral Manifestations of Grief and Recommended Nursing Interventions

Grief Behaviors	Nurse Behaviors (Recommended Nursing Interventions)
DENIAL (Shock)	
Verbal expression ("no, not me; it's not happening")	Allows initial denial
Shock, disbelief	Allows privacy
Inability to talk about loss	Encourages person to talk
Detachment and isolation	Facilitates emotional expression
Intellectualization of the loss	Allows and even encourages the presence of significant others
Mood swings	Accepts mood swings
	Offers comfort and support warranted by reality and the nature of the loss
ANGER (Awareness)	
Verbal expression	Encourages and accepts expression of feelings (anger)
Nonverbal communication	Stays with person and accepts inappropriate outlets
Physical expression	Encourages significant others to accept some "crazy behavior" from the person for a while
Projection of anger on others	Allows and even encourages crying
Inappropriate demands	Understands fearfulness
Emotional outbursts	Structures environment for as much support and constancy as possible
Crying	Encourages talking about loss
Agitation-irritability	
Fearfulness	
Expression of helplessness-hopelessness	
High anxiety	

SEARCHING (Relinquishment)

Guilt, regret ("If only I'd . . .")

Bringing up and talking about memories, images of lost object

Beginning to ask questions

Constantly reminding one's self that loss is real (permanent)

Looking for a previous experience (person, object)

Expecting the person lost to return at any minute

Taking on some of the behaviors of the person lost

Exploring similar experiences or talking with others who have undergone similar losses

Encourages and allows new behaviors when readiness for them is evident

Provides information about new activities

Emphasizes with profoundness and intensity of feelings and person's desire to have done something

Supports contact with others who have undergone similar losses

Avoids false reassurance

Provides encouragement

Allows talk and other realistic behavior associated with loss

REINVESTMENT (Resolution)

Active involvement with new interests

Reestablishment of friends

Planning for changes

Initiating activities and contacts

Sharing with others

Attempting to continue plans or activities of lost person in some way, perhaps through direct behaviors, benevolent contributions, or other symbolic actions

Encourages renewed interest in activities

Promotes future planning

Increases self-esteem, supports problem solving

Supports person's attempt to continue memories of lost one

Supports and even encourages independence

Prepares person for other difficult times for grief, such as anniversaries, holidays, and other times of special significance

Remains available for continued support as needed

normal life processes and conditions. Those life processes are the areas that most need nursing interventions from the perspective of the science of caring. They are also thought to be turning points between health and illness for the individual and the family. Since people now seek health more and more, nursing must also seek health. Knowledge, intervention, and research related to the three conditions and life processes of stress-change, developmental conflicts, and loss may help nursing as the science of caring by contributing to the scientific understanding of the psychosocial aspects of the delivery of health care.

REFERENCES

1. Biscof, L. J. *Adult Psychology.* New York: Harper & Row, 1969.
2. Bishop, A. Culture Shock Still Confronts Vietnamese. *The Denver Post,* March 29, 1977. P. 43.
3. Dohrenwend, B. S., and Dohrenwend, B. P. *Stressful Life Events.* New York: Wiley, 1974.
4. Engel, G. *Psychological Development in Health and Disease.* Philadelphia: Saunders, 1963.
5. Engel, G. Grief and grieving. *American Journal of Nursing* 64:93, 1964.
6. Erikson, E. *Childhood and Society* (2nd ed.). New York: Norton, 1963.
7. Erikson, E. *Identity: Youth and Crisis.* New York: Norton, 1968.
8. Freedman, A. M., Kaplan, H. I., and Sedock, B. J. *Modern Synopsis of Comprehensive Text of Psychiatry.* Baltimore: Williams & Wilkins, 1972.
9. Freud, S. (1917). *Mourning and Melancholia.* Complete Works Vol. 14 (Standard edition). London: Hogarth, 1953.
10. Freud, S. Grieving for a Lost Home. In L. Duhl (ed.), *The Urban Condition.* New York: Basic Books, 1963.
11. Glaser, B. G., and Strauss, A. *Awareness of Dying.* Chicago: Aldine, 1966.
12. Holmes, T. H., and Rahe, R. H. The social readjustment rating scale. *Journal of Psychosomatic Research* 11:213, 1967.
13. Howard, D. Vietnamese Resettlement. (Paper written to fulfill course requirement.) Denver, Colo.: University of Colorado School of Nursing. May, 1977.
14. Lindamann, E. Symptomatology and management of acute grief. *American Journal of Psychiatry* 101:141, 1944.
15. Marris, P. *Loss and Change.* New York: Random House, 1974.

16. Parkes, C. M. *Bereavement.* New York: International Universities Press, 1973.
17. Schoenberg, B., Carr, A., Peretz, D., and Kutscher, A. *Loss and Grief: Psychological Management in Medical Practice.* New York: Columbia University Press, 1970.
18. Schoenberg, B., Gerber, I., Wiener, A., et al. (eds.). *Bereavement: Its Psychosocial Aspects.* New York: Columbia Press, 1975.
19. Sheehy, G. *Passages.* New York: Dutton, 1976.
20. Turning Off the Last Lights: Evacuation. *Time,* May 5, 1975. Pp. 19–20.
21. Watson, J. Module on Loss of Self. In Loss Series, F. L. Bower (ed.). New York: Wiley. In press.

14. STRESS: HEALTH INTERVENTIONS RELATED TO STRESS; THE INDIVIDUAL'S PERCEPTIONS OF STRESS; WAYS OF COPING WITH STRESS; SITUATIONAL SUPPORTS FOR THE PERSON UNDER STRESS

Part III of this text has identified three major forces that are related to higher order concepts of health or wellness: (1) stress input (e.g., change), (2) developmental conflicts, and (3) loss. Quality of living is dependent to some degree on coping with those normal processes.

Those three processes are important for health interventions in that nursing care can incorporate them into the assessment, management, and evaluation of health care, "before the fact" of illness. Interventions that are systematically designed to promote health in a broad sense can begin by organizing care around the situations in daily life that require coping. Those common situations are change, developmental conflicts, and loss. Each situation is considered stressful, and it requires on-going coping. Each can be a turning point toward illness or health and a higher level of wellness, depending on the perception, coping mechanism, and situational supports of the person undergoing stress.

The nurse can intervene with another person at any time during illness, health, or wellness — and thus promote health.

NURSING HEALTH INTERVENTIONS
The nursing health interventions include the following:

1. *Examining the Total Person Context.* Where does the person see himself or herself on the continuum of illness-health-wellness (according to Travis's Wellness Scale)? A personal

Table 14-1. Psychiatrically Oriented Personal and Social History

Information	Syndromes or Conditions Relevant to Information
Upbringing	
1. Family constellation: intact or broken home—reasons if latter; number, age, and sex of siblings	Hysteria
2. Socioeconomic status of family	Antisocial personality
3. Religion—kind and importance in life	Problem traits
4. Discipline or nervous problems as child	
School history	
1. Highest grade attained	Mental retardation
2. Age stopped school—reasons	Antisocial personality
3. Academic performance: failed subjects, held back, special education, special interests	Problem traits
4. Discipline problems in school: suspended, expelled—reasons	
5. Extracurricular activities	
6. Adjustment—friends; attitude toward school	
Work history	
1. Type and number of jobs	Mental retardation, antisocial personality
2. Reasons for leaving jobs	
3. Inability to perform on jobs— reasons	Problem traits
4. Ever fired from jobs—reasons	Alcoholism or other drug dependency
5. Job satisfaction: plans and prospects for advancement	
Military history	
1. Branch of service and type of duties	Alcoholism or drug dependency; antisocial personality; problem traits
2. Any disciplinary action—reasons and outcome of difficulty in service	Above conditions plus schizophrenia, mental retardation, depression, etc.
3. Type of discharge: if other than honorable—reasons	
4. If *no* service, reasons for not serving	

Table 14-1 (continued)

Information	Syndromes or Conditions Relevant to Information
Sexual history 1. Sexual experience and education: first experiences, how learned, attitude toward sex 2. Homosexual experiences— circumstances and frequency 3. Specific problems with sexual performance or worries about sex 4. Family and personal attitudes toward sex 5. Pattern of sexual activity: number and kinds of partners (promiscuity)	Sexual variants, problem traits (e.g., excessive worry over masturbation); antisocial personality
Marital history 1. Number of marriages and reasons for divorces or separations 2. Physical and mental health problems in spouse 3. Present satisfaction with marriage 4. If single, reasons for not marrying	Alcoholism, antisocial personality, problem traits, schizophrenia
Premorbid personality (usual personality before mental or physical illness) 1. Social activities: friends, dating, clubs, including frequency and satisfaction with contacts 2. Interests and hobbies 3. Special abilities 4. Philosophy of life, including religious activities and affiliations 5. Personal habits: neatness, concern about appearance, drinking, smoking	Antisocial personality, problem traits, schizophrenia

Source: Cadoret and King [1].

Table 14-2. Flow of Thought and Speech

Behavior or Symptom	Description—How to Observe	Clinical Example
"Push of speech"	Note spontaneous production by patients of answers to questions; *try* to interrupt patient's conversation with a question; patients with "push" are hard to interrupt	In mania "push" is common; patient will often talk spontaneously without being questioned; rate of speech may be speeded
"Flight of ideas"	Note spontaneous production by patient of answers to questions; thought shows a rapid digression from one idea to another; connected train of thought usually apparent	Hallmark of mania. Question: How did you get here? Answer: My brother brought me in his car. He likes to drive. Cars are very expensive and I want to buy one. I like to shop a lot, don't you? When are you going to let me out so I can go to a store?
"Tangential" speech sometimes called "looseness of associations"; extreme degree of tangential speech termed "word salad"	Note spontaneous production of answers to questions; speech difficult or impossible to follow logically; connection between ideas not understandable	Question: How did you get here? Answer: My brother had a car. The weather is very good. When am I going to get out of here?
"Circumstantial"*	Note spontaneous production of answers to questions; overinclusion of many trivial and unnecessary details; person usually returns to the point and questions are eventually answered	Question: How did you get here? Answer: My brother said you better go to the hospital so I said to him, "You think so." He said "Yes" so I got my hat and then he said, "Wait a minute," so then I said, etc., etc.

Table 14-2 (continued)

Behavior or Symptom	Description—How to Observe	Clinical Example
Mute*	No verbal response to questions or spontaneous speech	Occurs in wide variety of conditions from organic brain syndrome to schizophrenia
Blocking*	Occurs spontaneously during interview; sudden stoppage of speech for few seconds to minutes without apparent external reason; train of thought often lost; might be nonresponsive during episode to usual stimuli	Schizophrenics sometimes complain of this happening to them; will describe spells when thoughts are taken away, or mind made blank ("thought stealing")

*Indicates nondiagnostic behavior.
Source: Cadoret and King [1].

Table 14-3. Psychiatrically Oriented Family History

Parents and Siblings	Family Interaction

For each individual determine:
1. Age and occupation
2. Personality—how close to patient
3. Present and past mental health (if dead, cause); assess by inquiry:
  a. "Nervous breakdowns" and their character, treatment, and whether recovered
  b. Suicide attempts and suicide
  c. Alcoholism or other drug dependency
  d. Psychiatric hospitalization or outpatient treatment
  e. Need for "tranquilizers," antidepressants, sedatives, or drugs for "nerves"
	1. Who lives at home or with patient
	2. Responsibilities and duties in home of different members of family, including patient
	3. How other members get along with each other and with patient
	4. How decisions are made which affect family or patient
	5. How discipline is carried out and its effectiveness
	6. Special problems: financial, illness in siblings or parents, crowded living conditions, interfering relatives, etc.

Source: Cadoret and King [1].

Table 14-4. Mental Status: General Appearance and Behavior

Behavior or Symptom	Description—How to Observe	Clinical Example
Grooming, general appearance	Compare appearance with social norm for patient	Bizarre bright-colored clothes with manics; slovenly appearance with food-stained clothing in persons with organic brain syndrome
Facial expression: angry, sad, anxious, puzzled, perplexed, tearful, etc.	Observation during interview—compare with usual social norms; facial expression important to assess ongoing affect and relate it to content of conversation (see Table 5)	Depressed individuals often look sad or pained, unhappy or tearful Manic often smiling, laughing boisterously
Motor activity: retarded (underactive), overactive; increased and decreased time between question and response	Compare speed of movements and reaction time to questions to "normal" for patient; note amount of *spontaneous* speech and movement	Slowness of movement and speech in depression; increased latency of response to questions in depression; rapid speech, movement, and quickness of response in mania
Level of consciousness: alert, confused, somnolent	Compare response to examiner and environment: *Alert*—normal attention to environment *Confused*—behavior suggests patient less able to recognize and understand environment *Somnolent*—tends to drift off to sleep when external stimuli cease; can be roused	May vary over time, especially in organic brain syndrome where fluctuating level of consciousness is a characteristic of certain conditions such as subdural hematoma

Source: Cadoret and King [1].

Table 14-5. Mental Status: Affect

Behavior or Symptom	Description—How to Observe	Clinical Example
Affect or mood	Affect is predominant emotional feeling over period of time; term mood is sometimes used interchangeably, though connotations of mood are for shorter-lived or more transient affective states	Can use such description as: "Affect was depressed" or "Mood was euphoric"
Depressed affect or mood	Note spontaneous appearance: sad facies, tearfulness Questions: How do you feel about the future? How are your spirits? How has your mood been lately?	Depressed individuals might describe mood as "down," "disgusted and fed up," "discouraged," "blue," "depressed," "unhappy," "black future," or "there is no future"
Elevated affect or mood (euphoria)	Note spontaneous appearance: happy facies, cheerful Question: How is your mood?	Manic individuals might describe mood as "up," "high," "euphoric," "great," "never felt better," "full of pep," "nothing bothers me"
Grandiose or expansive affect or mood	Note spontaneous appearance: may seem haughty, condescending Questions: Do you feel you have special abilities? Do you have exciting ideas, special powers or talents? Tell me about them.	Grandiose individuals such as some schizophrenics or especially manics might admit special abilities, mission in life, or powers from God
Other affects: perplexity; puzzlement; suspicion; hostility	Note spontaneous appearance: confused, bewildered, puzzled, or suspicious and angry	Perplexity and puzzlement found in schizophreniform syndrome; suspicion is the hallmark of schizophrenics of paranoid type who feel persecuted

Table 14-5 (continued)

Behavior or Symptom	Description—How to Observe	Clinical Example
Appropriate affect*	Observation of affect relative to topics discussed during interview; mood matches content of thought as expressed in the interview	Depressed person may be very self-depreciatory and unhappy
Inappropriate affect*	Mood does not match content of interview Question: How do you feel about the persecution you have undergone?	Schizophrenic might cry as he or she tells of happy event or laugh in silly manner about tragedy; some hysterics describe crippling and serious medical symptoms, such as paralyses with seeming indifferent ("la belle indifference")
Flattened affect*	Compare emotional display to what one would ordinarily expect as natural with change of topics during interview; very little modulation of affect with change of topics	Supposed to be hallmark of schizophrenic condition. When present appears as a "wooden" or "stony-faced" appearance similar to the facies of parkinsonism (in individuals on phenothiazines, may be difficult to distinguish from drug-induced parkinsonism)
Labile mood*	Observe changes of mood with topics or with external stimuli; mood changes easily with minimal stimulation or occurs spontaneously	

*Indicates nondiagnostic behavior.
Source: Cadoret and King [1].

social history, family history, and mental status assessment
are also valuable references for understanding the person.
Tables 14-1 to 14-5 provide a useful framework for con-
ducting an assessment interview that helps to "get at" the
total-person context for health promotion interventions.

2. *Determining What the Person Identifies as His or Her Stress
Inputs — Past, Present, and Future.* Those stresses may be
(a) *changes,* which can be measured by the Social Readjustment Rating Scale (see p. 85) and, more specifically, by
the changes that accompany the current situation, such as
injury or illness and health changes; (b) *developmental*
conflicts, which can be determined by knowledge of the
age of the patient and the psychosocial conflicts and developmental tasks that are associated with that age. A comprehensive health history, social family history, and a
psychosocial assessment that includes mental processes
(such as the patient's perceptions, prevailing mood,
thoughts, and the meaning of events to him or her) can
also be used. A study of developmental conflicts can use
the total-person context (see No. 1 in this list and Tables
14-1 to 14-5); or (c) *loss,* which can be studied with the
Social Readjustment Rating Scale (see p. 85). The life-
change score of a person tested with the Social Readjustment Rating Scale indicates how well the person is readjusting after his or her loss. Loss can be studied from the
perspectives of psychological losses, sociocultural losses,
and physical losses of the past, present, and future. Examples of such losses are losses associated with developmental
stages, such as marriage, pregnancy, starting or ending a job,
illness, or surgery. Certainly on top of those kinds of loss is
the profound loss of a significant other.

3. *Assessing the Person's Perception of the Stressful Event in
His or Her Own Life.* Perceptions can be assessed by ask-
ing how the person sees and understands the changes, conflicts, and losses that are taking place or that are anticipated.
Is the stress perceived as a threat or a loss — or as a challenge or a growth experience? Depending on the accuracy
and nature of the perceptions, the nursing intervention is
concentrated on (a) regulating the perception or (b) altering

the perception. The carative factor promotion of interpersonal teaching-learning is most effective as one form of
intervention related to perceptions. A variety of cognitive,
affective, and behavioral approaches may be used by the
nurse, one at a time or in combination, to promote accurate, realistic perceptions. Those approaches include (a)
giving cognitive information, (b) forming a relationship
with the patient in which he or she feels free to express his
or her emotions, (c) the nurse can encourage the patient to
engage in certain behaviors to alter his or her perceptions
(e.g., relaxation techniques, biofeedback, taking the patient
through a trial procedure before actually employing it, i.e.,
visiting a hospital room and meeting the hospital's staff
before the patient is hospitalized. Skill in the carative factor development of a helping-trust relationship is important in assessing perceptions.

4. *Promoting Constructive Coping Mechanisms.* While gather-
ing data about the stressful events in a person's life, the
nurse can assess the person's ways of coping with previous
change, loss, and developmental conflicts. Does the person
seek additional information in order to cope with stress?
Does the person act directly to alter a troubled transaction
between himself or herself and the environment? Is the
person inhibited in acting (e.g., does he or she feel helpless-
hopeless in manipulating the environment)? Does the person engage in intrapsychic processes that facilitate coping
(e.g., clarifying distortions, talking to himself or herself
mentally rehearsing a stressful event, altering the meaning
of a situation to make it a challenge instead of a threat)?
All these methods of coping tell the nurse about the person's pattern of coping and about what works and does
not work for him or her. Intervention can be based on
the person's pattern of coping and behaving. The interventions that best promote constructive coping are those
that assist the individual according to his or her strengths
and weaknesses.

5. *Promoting Situational Supports.* The nurse intervenes in
that area directly and indirectly. A nurse should find out
what situational supports are present or absent in order to

intervene effectively. What support do the family, friends, colleagues, peers, and co-workers of the patient give him or her? What socioeconomic, physical, emotional, and behavioral resources does the environment give the patient? What health care delivery system supports does the patient have? What social services and other types of services does the patient have access to? Last, how can the nurse and nursing care be situational supports? The range of possibilities extends from structuring the patient's physical environment to encouraging the family to develop a better relationship with the patient.

All the nursing interventions in the science of caring that are designed to promote health and a higher level of wellness can be organized to help a person deal with common stress situations, the person's perceptions of the event, his or her patterns of coping, and the situational supports available to him or her. Health can be promoted through the carative factors discussed in this text. Interventions can be cognitive, affective, or behavioral, or they can be a combination of those activities. Depending on the nature of the illness-health-wellness phenomenon for a person, the stressful life events (change, conflict, loss) he or she undergoes, his or her ways of coping, and situational supports, the nurse orders interventions that are best for the particular person; that is, interventions designed to promote accurate, realistic perceptions, coping that leads to constructive action and situational supports.

The figure on page 302 illustrates the process of stressful life events that can lead either to illness or to health promotion and illness prevention. The model gives a background of past experiences, situational supports, and previous and present ways of coping that affect a person's responses to current stressful events in life.

The heavy black lines represent major life changes, severe developmental conflicts, and profound loss. The lighter black lines represent moderately stressful events; and the thin dotted lines represent slightly stressful events. The stressful event's magnitude evokes psychological-behavioral responses and biophysical responses that attempt to lessen the magnitude of the

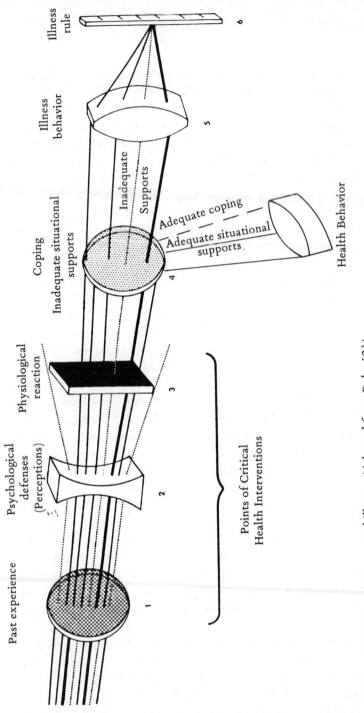

Past experience

Psychological defenses (Perceptions)

Physiological reaction

Coping

Inadequate situational supports

Inadequate Supports

Adequate coping

Adequate situational supports

Health Behavior

Illness behavior

Illness rule

Points of Critical Health Interventions

Pathway between stress input and illness. (Adapted from Rahe [2]) stress. Intense coping results from the stressful events. Maintaining health or the onset of illness depends on (1) past stressful experiences and coping, (2) current coping-adapting, and (3) the intervention of health professionals, as well as other situational supports. Depending on the coping and the interventions, the stress response can lead to (1) inadequate coping, perceptions, situational supports, illness behaviors, and illness onset (physical or psychological) or (2) coping, wellness behaviors, and health maintenance and illness prevention.

Coping is a dynamic, evolving, unending process that tries to maintain a balanced relationship between the individual and the environment. Specific types of interventions help persons to cope effectively in a given environment. Among the interventions are:

1. Assessment of the stressful events.
2. Self-exploration and awareness of the subjective importance of the events. The philosophy of internal control over one's life is a factor. The accuracy of one's perceptions and the meaning of the event (threat, harm, loss, or challenge) can be critical.
3. Minimizing the stress of the events; for example, by changing one's life-style and pace of living, being more careful about safety, anticipating developmental conflicts, effectively resolving loss, making changes in one's job, getting enough exercise, concentrating on tasks, engaging in activities that bring self-satisfaction, relaxation, fulfillment of one's goals, release of physical and emotional energy and fulfillment of basic needs (e.g., nutrition-elimination, activity-inactivity — rest/work/play — achievement, affiliation, sexuality, ventilation-respiration, and the movement toward self-awareness and self-actualization).
4. The promotion of adequate ways of coping includes the interventions just mentioned, and it supports quality of life and health professional caring responses in a human-to-human relationship. The promotion of ways of coping includes the acknowledgment of feelings (positive and negative ones), allowing the person to express anger, joy, pain, sorrow and love, and supporting him or her when he or she

does so; helping to alter the troubled transactions between a person and his or her environment or changing the meaning of stress from threat to challenge.

5. If coping mechanisms are not supported, promoted, or channeled at the stress-coping point, the person may then develop inadequate coping because of (a) his or her past experiences and maladaptive strategies, (b) the nature of the stressful events, or (c) inadequate health intervention from the health professionals concerned with primary health care delivery. At a later point, the coping mechanisms may need to be corrected through either medical or psychological intervention-treatment. Even so, illness behaviors and the onset of illness become more likely. A person showing illness behaviors pays attention to the symptoms of illness (either psychological or physical illness) and seeks medical treatment. The person's symptoms are diagnosed as pathological and indicative of illness.

In this text, health is presented in a broad context of the quality of life, which includes the perception of and coping with stressful life events. In that context the nursing interventions necessary to promote health and prevent illness are identified. The conceptual model in the figure on page 302 shows how psychological, social, and physical factors affect stressful life events and in turn require primary preventive interventions.

Recent evidence indicates that persons who handle stress with good psychological defense mechanisms may keep stresses from affecting them physically. Health interventions should occur at the beginning of the lens model. Health professionals who deliver primary care must consider the broader areas of health and life if health is to be promoted. Helping others to gain control over their patterns of coping and stressful life events may be the ultimate health intervention — one that not only prevents illness but also promotes a higher quality of life and a higher level of wellness.

SUMMARY
Many theories, concepts, research findings, and perspectives have been presented in this text. The text's goal is to provide

a structure for studying and understanding nursing as the science of caring. The carative factors discussed in this text are the knowledge and professional forces the nurse should bring to all human transactions. Those carative factors can be translated into organized instrumental or expressive nursing interventions. Holistic health, stressful life events, and a nursing health intervention framework form an overall closing perspective for the text. Much of the material has focused on the psychosocial aspects of caring. The parameters provide a tentative foundation for nursing as the science of caring, and they need to be further delineated, studied and researched. The goal of such study is the development of a body of philosophical and scientific knowledge that helps a nurse care for another person before, during, and after illness.

REFERENCES

1. Cadoret, R. J., and King, L. J. *Psychiatry in Primary Care.* St. Louis: Mosby, 1974. Pp. 16–21.
2. Rahe, R. Pathway Between Subjects' Recent Life Changes and Their Near-Future Illness Reports: Representative Results and Methodological Issues. In B. S. Dohrenwend and B. P. Dohrenwend (eds.), *Stressful Life Events.* New York: Wiley, 1974. P. 75.

INDEX

INDEX

Achievement, 175–183; activity need and, 153, 156–157; expectations and, 179–180, 180–181, 182, 183; goal of, 175; motivation and, 175–176, 177, 181, 182; need, defined, 175; origin and development of need in children, 176–177, 178, 182; psychological factors and, 181–182; self-actualization and, 175; sexual differences in motivation for, 170, 177; significance of need for practice of caring, 181, 182–183; social learning theory applied to, 178–179; sociocultural factors and, 175, 178, 179, 180–181, 182; value systems and, 180, 182

Ackerknecht, E. H., quoted, 14

Action in coping, 260

Action level communication, described, 33

Activity-inactivity: achievement and self-actualization and, 153, 156–157; changes in, effects of, 147–148, 149, 150; constructive and nonconstructive features of, 148–149; dimensions in continuum of energy utilization, 146–147; energy channelization, 148–150; environmental change and, 150; fatigue and boredom, 161, 162; fundamental vital nature of, 145; gratification of need, 146–147, 150, 155–157, 161; importance of constructive, 151; psychological

factors and, 148, 149–150, 151–155, 156, 163; rest, 158, 160–161, 162; significance in practice of caring, 162–163; sleep, 157–160, 162–163; sociocultural factors and, 148–149

Adaptation: emotions associated with, 117; to loss, 273, 282–285, 286–287; need gratification and, 107

Adler, A., 13, 189, 199

Affect. See Emotions

Affection, need for, 186

Affiliation need, 183–192; basic nature and function of, 184, 186; environment and development of affiliation system, 185, 187, 188, 191; expression and behavior and, 186–188, 191; family group and, 188, 191; as foundation for relationships, 184, 191; health-illness changes and, 189–190, 191–192; humanism and, 183–184, 191; interpersonal needs and, 185–186, 187, 191; models of behaviors expressing, 189, 191; origin and development of affiliative behavior, 184–185, 187, 188, 191; significance for practice of caring, 191–192; social group experiences and, 187–188, 191

Alexander, F., 120

Allport, G. W., quoted, 12

Altruism. See Humanistic-altruistic value system

American Academy of Nursing, 239

Anorexia nervosa, 118, 121

Appley, M. H., 70

Appraisal, as clinical care phase, 77